The Maudsley® Prescribing Guidelines for Mental Health Conditions in Physical Illness

T0337865

THE MAUDSLEY® GUIDELINES

Other books in the *Maudsley® Prescribing Guidelines* series include:

The Maudsley® Prescribing Guidelines in Psychiatry, 14th Edition
David M. Taylor, Thomas R. E. Barnes, Allan H. Young

The Maudsley® Practice Guidelines for Physical Health Conditions in Psychiatry
David M. Taylor, Fiona Gaughran, Toby Pillinger

The Maudsley® Guidelines on Advanced Prescribing in Psychosis
Paul Morrison, David M. Taylor, Phillip McGuire

The Maudsley® Deprescribing Guidelines: Antidepressants, Benzodiazepines, Gabapentinoids and Z-drugs
Mark Horowitz, David M. Taylor

The Maudsley® Prescribing Guidelines for Mental Health Conditions in Physical Illness

Siobhan Gee, MPharm, PGDip, MRPharmS (consultant), PhD

Consultant Pharmacist and Deputy Director of Pharmacy, South London and the Maudsley NHS Foundation Trust
Honorary Senior Lecturer, King's College, London, UK

David M. Taylor, BSc, MSc, PhD, FFRPS, FRPharmS, FRCP$_{Edin}$, FRCPsych(Hon)

Director of Pharmacy and Pathology, South London and Maudsley NHS Foundation Trust
Professor of Psychopharmacology, King's College, London, UK

WILEY Blackwell

This edition first published 2025
© 2025 John Wiley & Sons Ltd

Registered Offices
John Wiley & Sons, Inc., 111 River Street, Hoboken, NJ 07030, USA
John Wiley & Sons Ltd, The Atrium, Southern Gate, Chichester, West Sussex, PO19 8SQ, UK

For details of our global editorial offices, customer services, and more information about Wiley products visit us at www.wiley.com.

Wiley also publishes its books in a variety of electronic formats and by print-on-demand. Some content that appears in standard print versions of this book may not be available in other formats.

Library of Congress Cataloging-in-Publication Data is applied for

Paperback ISBN: 9781394192403

Cover Design: Wiley

Set in 10/12pt Sabon by Straive, Pondicherry, India

SKY10090858_111324

Contents

Preface

More than 40% of people diagnosed with a serious mental illness have at least one concurrent physical illness. Prescribing medicines to treat the psychiatric condition can be complex in these circumstances. The prescriber will need to consider both the potential for prescribed medication to adversely affect any physical health condition and the possibility of altered response because of the presence of physical illness. Choice of medication in the physically unwell patient can be further complicated by a host of other factors. Some patients, for example, cannot take medicines orally, some are at the end of life, some may be on renal replacement therapy, and so on.

The challenges of managing mental health medicines in patients with complex physical comorbidity are faced daily in liaison psychiatry (also known as consultative psychiatry or consultation-liaison psychiatry). As the global population ages and the prevalence of psychiatric conditions continues to increase, these challenges are also increasingly faced by psychiatrists working in all specialisms, both acute and chronic, inpatient and outpatient. This book aims to help the clinician navigate these prescribing scenarios and to be of use not only to psychiatrists but general physicians too.

The importance of treating psychiatric conditions in people with physical illness cannot be overstated. There is no doubt that for every physical illness, the presence of mental ill health adversely affects both morbidity and mortality. We hope this book will not only enable the choice of safe and effective medication in physically unwell patients, but also engender confident prescribing for mental illness, even in the face of severe physical illness.

Siobhan Gee
David M. Taylor
July 2024

Acknowledgements

The following have contributed to the 1st edition of the *Maudsley® Prescribing Guidelines for Mental Health Conditions in Physical Illness*.

John Archer
Grainne D'Ancona
Mary-Jane Docherty
Petrina Douglas-Hall
Alexa Duff
Nicola Kalk
Cathrine McKenzie
Calum Moulton
Larissa Ryan
Mark Samaan
Esha Sharma
Clare Thomson
Jessica Webb
Hayley Wells

Particular thanks go to colleagues based within the Mind & Body Programme at King's Health Partners who obtained funding from the Maudsley Charity in 2019 to facilitate the development of these guidelines. The work of the Mind & Body Programme continues at King's Health Partners to provide integrated mental and physical healthcare that aims to improve care and outcomes for patients in South East London. For more information, please contact mindandbody@slam.nhs.uk.

Abbreviations

ACE	angiotensin-converting enzyme
ADHD	attention deficit hyperactivity disorder
APD	automated peritoneal dialysis
ARF	acute respiratory failure
ATP	adenosine triphosphate
BD	bis die (twice a day)
BMI	body mass index
BNP	B-type natriuretic peptide
BP	blood pressure
cAMP	cyclic adenosine monophosphate
CAPD	continuous ambulatory peritoneal dialysis
CCV	central compartment volume
CHD	coronary heart disease
CNS	central nervous system
COPD	chronic obstructive pulmonary disorder
CRP	C-reactive protein
CYP	cytochrome P
DSM-5	*Diagnostic and Statistical Manual 5*
ECG	electrocardiogram
ECHO	echocardiogram
ECT	electroconvulsive therapy
ENRICHD	enhancing recovery in coronary heart disease
EPSE	extrapyramidal side effect
FBC	full blood count
FDA	Food and Drug Administration
GABA	gamma-aminobutyric acid
GI	gastrointestinal
HDAC9	histone deacetylase 9
IBD	inflammatory bowel disease
ICS	inhaled corticosteroid
ICU	intensive care unit
IL	interleukin
IM	intramuscular

INR	international normalised ratio
IV	intravenous
LABA	long-acting beta-2 agonist
LAMA	long-acting muscarinic antagonist
MAO	monoamine oxidase
MAOI	monoamine oxidase inhibitor
MDMA	3,4-methylenedioxymethamphetamine
MI	myocardial infarction
MIND-IT	myocardial infarction and depression intervention trial
MOOD-HF	mood and mortality in depressed heart failure patients
NaCl	sodium chloride
NaSSA	noradrenaline and specific serotonergic antidepressant
NG	nasogastric
NHS	National Health Service
NICE	National Institute for Health and Care Excellence
NJ	nasojejunal
NMDA	N-methyl-d-aspartate
NNT	number needed to treat
NOAC	non-vitamin K antagonist oral anticoagulant
NRT	nicotine replacement therapy
NSAID	non-steroidal anti-inflammatory drug
NT-pro BNP	N-terminal pro B-type natriuretic peptide
OD	omni die (once a day)
PEG	percutaneous endoscopic gastrostomy
QTc	QT interval adjusted for heart rate
RASS	Richmond Agitation Sedation Scale
RCT	randomised controlled trial
SABA	short-acting beta-2 agonist
SADHART-CHF	sertraline against depression and heart disease in chronic heart failure
SAMA	short-acting muscarinic antagonist
SC	subcutaneous
SIADH	syndrome of inappropriate antidiuretic hormone secretion
SL	sublingual
SMI	serious mental illness
SNRI	serotonin and noradrenaline reuptake inhibitor
SSRI	selective serotonin reuptake inhibitor
STAR*D	Sequenced Treatment Alternatives to Relieve Depression programme
TCA	tricyclic antidepressant
TDS	ter die sumendum (three times a day)
TNF	tumour necrosis factor
UC	ulcerative colitis
UK	United Kingdom
USA	United States of America
Vd	volume of distribution

Chapter 1

Cardiac Disease

CONTENTS

The Maudsley® Prescribing Guidelines for Mental Health Conditions in Physical Illness, First Edition.
Siobhan Gee and David M. Taylor.
© 2025 John Wiley & Sons Ltd. Published 2025 by John Wiley & Sons Ltd.

INTRODUCTION

The influence of psychiatric symptoms on the functioning of the heart was first described in 1628 by Sir William Harvey, the English physician who discovered the cardiac circulatory system. Since then, numerous studies have proven him correct, finding mental illness to be a significant predictor of cardiac mortality across the spectrum of cardiac diseases. Treatment of the mental illness is therefore vital not only for relief of psychiatric symptoms, but also for optimal treatment of the cardiac disease.

Few data are available to compare efficacy of drugs for mental illness within individual physical illnesses, such as heart failure or coronary heart disease, and even fewer for patients who have more than one concurrent physical illness. When extrapolating data from studies in patients without cardiac disease, it should be noted that populations studied in these trials are different (e.g. cardiac disease patients tend to be older than populations with general depression). Perhaps more importantly, the biological symptoms of mental illnesses that are measured by standard rating scales may not appear to improve on addition of psychiatric drugs because of the overlap of these physical symptoms with ongoing symptoms of the heart disease (e.g. fatigue, insomnia). Failure to demonstrate response to a drug on a rating scale is of little importance in clinical practice (symptoms are the target) but is relevant if trial data are used to make decisions about drug choice. Conversely, it is also possible that illnesses such as depression or anxiety – specifically in the context of heart disease – are biologically distinct from general depression. Consequently, drug treatments may not be effective for this reason.

HEART FAILURE

Depression and anxiety in heart failure

As many as one in five patients with heart failure suffer from depression, more than doubling the mortality risk and trebling the risk of non-compliance with medical treatment recommendations[1]. Clinically significant symptoms of anxiety are also commonly reported in patients with heart failure (30%)[2]. Symptoms of heart failure and those of anxiety may overlap, increasing the apparent prevalence. A clear link between anxiety and mortality in heart failure has not been fully established, but an increased risk is evident for patients with other cardiac disorders such as coronary artery disease[3]. Of course, depression and anxiety may co-exist, and together they increase the risk of both cardiac rehospitalisation and mortality in patients with heart failure[4].

There are several factors that may give rise to the link between depression and anxiety, and poor cardiac outcomes in heart failure. These include biological changes that occur in association with the mental health condition (inflammation, autonomic dysfunction, alterations in the ability of platelets to aggregate, and endothelial dysfunction[2]). Adherence to medicines for the treatment of the heart failure or comorbidities may be affected, as may maintenance of a healthy lifestyle (smoking cessation, diet, exercise).

There are few data relating to the efficacy of pharmacotherapy in depression specifically with comorbid heart failure. The most well-known studies are SADHART-CHF (Sertraline Against Depression and Heart Disease in Chronic Heart Failure) and MOOD-HF (Mood and Mortality in Depressed Heart Failure patients). SADHART-CHF demonstrated safety (although not efficacy) of sertraline[5], and MOOD-HF[6] the same for escitalopram. There are no randomised trials examining the pharmacological treatment of anxiety in heart failure patients.

Psychosis and bipolar disorder in heart failure

Patients with serious mental illness (SMI – schizophrenia, bipolar disorder, and severe depression) have a reduced life expectancy compared with the non-SMI population[7]. Cardiovascular disease is a significant contributor to this[8]. Lifestyle interventions are as important in this population as they are in the general population[9]. Antipsychotics and mood stabilisers (lithium and mood-stabilising antiepileptics) commonly cause weight gain, hyperglycaemia, and hyperlipidaemia. Despite this, patients who take them have an overall reduction in cardiac (and all-cause) mortality[10]. This may be a direct beneficial effect of reduction in psychiatric symptoms, improved adherence to healthy lifestyle choices, and/or better compliance with physical health treatments. Heart failure outcomes in patients who have SMI are therefore strongly linked to the outcome of their mental illness, making effective treatment of the psychiatric symptoms a priority. This is an important factor when weighing the risks and benefits of individual psychiatric medication choice. Medication that is perceived as safer in heart failure but less effective for the mental disorder may not actually be the optimal choice for overall cardiac outcomes[11].

Antidepressants

In general, SSRIs are considered first-line antidepressants, and this is also true for patients with heart failure. Of the SSRIs, sertraline[12,13] is generally well tolerated and efficacious in non-heart failure populations[14]. It has few drug interactions, less propensity than citalopram to prolong the QTc, and has been studied in patients with heart failure (it is safe, but efficacy is unproven)[5]. Escitalopram has also demonstrated safety (although not efficacy) in patients with heart failure[6], but is more often associated with QT prolongation[15] than sertraline (although this association is disputed[16]).

Other options carry some cautions. Mirtazapine is consistently shown to promote appetite, probably due to α_2 receptor blockade and affinity for H_1, D_1, and D_2 receptors[17], and is therefore less desirable in conditions such as heart failure where excess weight can be detrimental to clinical outcomes. Citalopram may be more likely than other antidepressants to prolong the QT interval and is not recommended for use in uncompensated heart failure[18]. SNRIs (venlafaxine and duloxetine) are associated with dose-dependent increases in blood pressure[19] (see section on hypertension), and venlafaxine and fluoxetine may also cause prolonged QT, particularly in combination with ivabradine[20]. Tricyclic antidepressants (TCAs) are generally avoided in patients with cardiac disease due to their effects on cardiac contractility, their proarrhythmic effects (due to blockade of cardiac sodium and potassium channels), and their potential to worsen ischaemic heart disease.

Hyponatraemia is a risk with all antidepressants in the first month of treatment. Depending on the patient's risk profile, the diuretic dose may need to be adjusted. If hyponatraemia persists, the dose of sacubitril may need to be reduced or stopped. Mirtazapine and agomelatine may be less commonly associated with hyponatraemia (but are not completely without risk). Close monitoring of sodium levels is recommended, especially in the first few weeks of treatment[21] and if patients have additional risk factors for developing hyponatraemia.

Recommendation: sertraline.

Antipsychotics

Most antipsychotics are associated to some degree with numerous cardiac adverse events, including prolonged QT interval, tachycardia and orthostatic hypotension. They can also (rarely) cause myocarditis and cardiomyopathy, which can lead to the development of heart failure. Pharmacovigilance studies suggest that myocarditis and cardiomyopathy may be particularly associated with chlorpromazine, fluphenazine, risperidone, and haloperidol (and clozapine; see below)[22]. Haloperidol, olanzapine, quetiapine, risperidone, and sulpiride have higher affinity than others for cardiac potassium channels and are associated with a higher risk of ventricular arrhythmia and sudden cardiac death[23]. Cariprazine, lurasidone, brexpiprazole, and lumateperone are considered safer choices in patients at risk of cardiac events, as they appear to exert minimal effects on the QT interval. They, along with 'typical' antipsychotics such as haloperidol, are also less likely than other 'atypical' drugs to cause weight gain and have adverse effects on blood lipids[24]. Olanzapine and clozapine are particularly problematic in this regard, and so may worsen the patient's cardiovascular risk factor profile.

Where patients develop symptomatic heart failure that is suspected to be caused by antipsychotic-induced cardiomyopathy, the offending drug should be changed to a different agent. For some patients this may be challenging if their psychiatric illness fails to respond to alternative antipsychotics. It has been suggested that a cut-off of 45% ejection fraction be used as a threshold for treatment cessation, extrapolating from guidelines for monitoring of cardiotoxic chemotherapies[25], but the exact level depends on the clinical scenario. After this point, studies indicate that the left ventricular function is less likely to recover[25]. Up to this threshold, effective antipsychotic treatments can be continued with 3-monthly monitoring of heart failure symptoms and NT-proBNP (a significant rise indicates raised cardiac filling pressures and should prompt an ECHO)[26].

For patients with pre-existing heart failure who require an antipsychotic, or need their current antipsychotic switched, choice of drug should primarily be focused on efficacy and tolerability. As described above, cariprazine, lurasidone, brexpiprazole, and lumateperone are preferable from a cardiac safety perspective. It is not known whether pre-existing heart failure predisposes to drug-induced cardiomyopathy, but it is the case that drug-induced cardiomyopathy worsens heart failure. For this reason, monitoring for any unexpected deterioration in cardiac function on commencing a new antipsychotic in someone with heart failure is recommended. Continued vigilance is required as antipsychotics may cause cardiomyopathy after many months of treatment, and this monitoring is best managed in a multidisciplinary setting involving both the psychiatry and cardiology teams.

Recommendation: cariprazine, lurasidone, brexpiprazole, lumateperone. Avoid olanzapine.

Clozapine

Of the antipsychotics, clozapine is particularly associated with myocarditis and cardiomyopathy (although these are still rare events). Nonetheless, it is possible to start clozapine in patients with pre-existing heart failure or continue clozapine if heart

CHAPTER 1

Table 1.1 Antipsychotics in heart failure

Event		Action
Antipsychotic-induced cardiomyopathy with symptoms of heart failure	Antipsychotic is effective.	Continue treatment if ejection fraction > 45%.
		Switch treatment if ejection fraction < 45%.
		Monitor symptoms and NT-proBNP 3 monthly.
	Antipsychotic is ineffective.	Switch, ideally to cariprazine, lurasidone, brexpiprazole, or lumateperone.
Non-antipsychotic induced heart failure (new or pre-existing)	Antipsychotic is effective.	Continue treatment.
	Antipsychotic is ineffective.	Switch, ideally to cariprazine, lurasidone, brexpiprazole, or lumateperone.
Antipsychotic-induced cardiomyopathy with ejection fraction < 45%. Offending antipsychotic has been stopped but alternative agents are ineffective.		Ensure optimisation of heart failure treatments before and during rechallenge. Ideally, wait until ejection fraction > 45%.
		Restart antipsychotic using a slow dose titration.
		Minimum weekly assessment of heart failure symptoms, HR, temp, trop, BNP, ECG[26] during dose titration (some authors suggest twice weekly troponin and CRP[28]).
		ECHO on completion of dose titration or earlier if indicated by symptoms or blood tests.

failure develops during treatment. In many cases this may be essential. Switching to a different antipsychotic when clozapine is indicated will almost inevitably result in psychiatric relapse. This can have dire consequences on the ability of the patient to comply with treatment for heart failure. Successful rechallenge with clozapine, even where cardiomyopathy is thought to be clozapine-induced, is achievable[27]. The enhanced risk of drug-induced cardiomyopathy with clozapine when compared with other antipsychotics means that monitoring cardiac function whilst establishing treatment is even more important. Use a slow titration of initial doses and monitor as described in Table 1.1.

Mood stabilisers

Pharmacovigilance database studies have linked lithium to an increased risk of myocarditis and cardiomyopathy[22], and case reports describe various cardiac adverse effects, including sinus node dysfunction, premature ventricular beats, atrioventricular block, and T-wave depression. These risks must be balanced against the (probably unparalleled) efficacy of lithium in bipolar disorder. Carbamazepine may be associated with hypotension, bradycardia, atrioventricular block, and possibly heart failure[29]. Heart failure has also been reported with valproate[30], and a Danish cohort study recently found an increased hazard ratio for mortality due to heart failure in elderly patients with epilepsy treated with valproate, compared with lamotrigine (or leveti-racetam)[31]. The authors postulated that this association may be due to the effect on cardiac conduction by valproate blockade of voltage-gated sodium channels, and possibly upregulation of anabolism of angiotensin II[31]. Other antiseizure drugs do not share this effect on angiotensin and may be safer.

In 2021, a warning that lamotrigine exhibits class 1B antiarrhythmic activity was added to the FDA product label. To date, no other regulatory authority has done the same. The warning is based on unpublished *in vitro* studies demonstrating that lamotrigine inhibits cardiac sodium channels, and may therefore slow ventricular condition, inducing arrhythmia. A study in healthy patients failed to find any such ECG changes, but it is possible that people with structural heart disease or myocardial ischaemia are at higher risk. Consequently, the FDA recommends avoiding lamotrigine in people who have cardiac conduction disorders, ventricular arrhythmias, or cardiac disease (including heart failure). The risk may be higher in people with elevated heart rates or who are taking other sodium channel blockers[32].

Recommendation: no drug is without risk. Lamotrigine may be preferable.

Others

Pregabalin can cause peripheral oedema, and case reports have been published reporting an associated with exacerbation of heart failure[29]. It should be used with caution, depending on the clinical scenario. **Promethazine** is a phenothiazine derivative and may prolong the QT interval, but the likelihood of progression to torsade de pointes appears to be low[33]. **Diphenhydramine** has been linked to QT prolongation in case reports, but in the context of congenital abnormalities[34] or overdose[35].

Benzodiazepines may worsen outcomes in heart failure. In two studies examining the management of insomnia[36] or anxiety[37] in heart failure, use of benzodiazepines was associated with increased rehospitalisation for heart failure and cardiovascular death. It is possible that this is a result of reduced respiratory drive adversely affecting heart failure symptoms. Conversely, a cohort study with an average 8-year follow-up period found a reduction in mortality for patients with heart failure prescribed benzodiazepines[38], perhaps reflecting the impact of improved management of mental health on heart failure outcomes. This is echoed by a multicentre Spanish study[39], where use of benzodiazepines during acute exacerbations of heart failure was not associated with differences in mortality after 7 days, despite patients receiving benzodiazepines having more severe cardiac symptoms at baseline. The dose may be important. A large Taiwanese study[40] found a reduction in cardiovascular mortality and hospitalisation for heart failure in patients receiving benzodiazepines post myocardial infarction, but only where small doses were used (up to 5mg diazepam, or equivalent). This benefit was lost at higher doses, possibly due to confounding by disease severity (higher doses implying higher levels of anxiety), or interference with cardiac rehabilitation.

Overall, it is clear that treatment of anxiety is important for cardiac outcomes, and benzodiazepines may be useful but should ideally be reserved for short-term use, in line with more general guidance on management of anxiety disorders.

The **cholinesterase inhibitors** (donepezil, rivastigmine, galantamine) can have vagotonic effects on the heart rate (i.e. bradycardia), and some cases of QT interval prolongation have been reported. These events are uncommon[41], and several studies show a protective effect of cholinesterase inhibitors on new-onset heart failure[42] or heart failure hospitalisation[43]. **Memantine** also appears to be safe in heart failure and may reduce hospitalisation[44].

CORONARY HEART DISEASE

Depression and anxiety in coronary heart disease

Between 15% and 30% of patients with coronary heart disease (CHD) are diagnosed with depression, a prevalence two to three times higher than the general population[45], and experts consider this to be an underestimation. Depression is a risk factor not only for the development of CHD but for cardiovascular morbidity and mortality in patients with established CHD[46]. Numerous mechanisms have been proposed to explain this relationship[47], both biological (altered autonomic nervous system activity, increased catecholamine levels, increased inflammatory activity, endothelial dysfunction, and platelet dysfunction) and behavioural (sedentary behaviour, poor diet, smoking, low medication adherence). There are now several studies examining whether treating depression can improve outcomes in CHD. The largest of these, ENRICHD[48], failed to find any reduction in cardiac events when sertraline was given to patients who had had a myocardial infarction. However, secondary analysis of this and other trials, including SADHART[49,50] and MIND-IT[51], suggests that improvement in depression may positively affect overall survival in patients with CHD.

Similarly, anxiety symptoms are common in CHD[52]. Anxiety is also an independent risk factor for the development of CHD[53], and for cardiac[54] and all-cause mortality[55] in CHD, particularly when comorbid with depression[55]. Despite this, there are very few studies specifically examining treatment of anxiety disorders as a primary outcome. Where they do exist, only generalised anxiety disorder or health-related anxiety are assessed (e.g. anxiety specifically around a cardiac intervention)[56]. Of note, anxiety disorders may share common symptoms with CHD, including tachycardia, shortness of breath, and chest pain.

Psychosis and bipolar disorder in coronary heart disease

A very large meta-analysis that included more than 3 million patients with serious mental illness and over 100 million controls[8] confirmed an increased risk of CHD for people with schizophrenia. There was no significant association between CHD and bipolar disorder in this analysis, but bipolar disorder has been significantly associated with cardiovascular disease in longitudinal studies, and with cardiovascular-related death[8].

Some data suggest that of the SMI subtypes, bipolar disorder confers the highest 10-year cardiovascular risk[57]. Various contributing factors are proposed, including accelerated atherosclerosis, endothelial dysfunction, and oxidative stress[58]. Despite the increased risk, patients with SMI are less likely to receive evidence-based management of CHD, both in terms of diagnosis and treatment[58].

Antidepressants

TCAs should be avoided in patients with CHD. Studies demonstrate negative cardiac outcomes for patients with CHD taking TCAs (increased heart rate, reduction in heart rate variability, and increased pulse[59,60]). The safety of SSRIs and mirtazapine post myocardial infarction (MI) has been demonstrated in several landmark studies[5,48,61], and it has further been suggested that the inhibitory effect of SSRIs on platelet activation may actually protect against MI[62]. This potential benefit (studies thus far have been underpowered to confirm this claim[5]) must be balanced against the increased risk of bleeding and gastric ulceration[63] when co-prescribing serotonergic antidepressants with aspirin or other antiplatelet therapies. A patient-centred approach is suggested – mirtazapine may be preferred over sertraline if the patient is felt to be at significant increased risk of bleeding, but balance this with the increased longer-term risk of weight gain with mirtazapine. See section on anticoagulation.

Recommendation: sertraline, or mirtazapine if significant bleeding risk.

Antipsychotics

Whether antipsychotics increase the risk of CHD is not clear. Some meta-analyses suggest an increased risk of MI for antipsychotic drug users[64,65], others do not[66,67]. The heterogeneity and retrospective design of many of the published studies (making it difficult to control for confounding factors) may be contributing to the variation in results. When considering individual antipsychotic drug choice, several factors may be relevant. These include the likelihood of the antipsychotic to cause ventricular arrhythmia (a cause of sudden cardiac death), or to prolong the QT interval (increasing the risk of torsades de pointes, leading to sudden cardiac death). The effect of the antipsychotic on metabolic parameters is also important, as cholesterol and triglyceride concentrations, hypertension, and obesity are associated with increased risk of CHD[68]. One study suggested that D_3 receptor antagonism may contribute to the development of MI, possibly because of effects on platelet aggregation, atherosclerosis, vascular remodelling, and intimal permeability[69]. The authors linked this to their observation that amisulpride, a drug with particularly high affinity for the D_3 receptor, also had the highest risk of MI in their study. This finding requires replication.

Antipsychotics with no apparent effect on the QT interval are cariprazine, brexpiprazole, lurasidone, and lumateperone[12], and these drugs also have more benign metabolic profiles than others[24]. They are therefore preferred in patients with CHD. Aripiprazole may be used if a depot is required (note that there is a possible association with QT interval prolongation[12]).

Recommendation: cariprazine, lurasidone, brexpiprazole, or lumateperone.

Mood stabilisers

Lithium can be used in CHD, with some data suggesting it may even slow the progression of atherosclerosis[70] and reduce cardiovascular mortality[71]. It can cause ECG changes, but at therapeutic plasma concentrations these are usually clinically insignificant[72] (but note that the manufacturers contraindicate lithium use in cardiac disorders with rhythm changes). Carbamazepine is an inducer of the hepatic cytochrome P450 enzyme system, which is involved in the synthesis of cholesterol. As a result, carbamazepine increases serum cholesterol[73,74] and this may translate to an increased risk of MI[75]. Lamotrigine and valproate do not negatively affect cholesterol concentrations[73]. Valproate is particularly associated with weight gain[73] but several studies show that use is associated with lower cholesterol concentrations, and possibly a corresponding reduction in the incidence of MI[75-77].

Recommendation: lithium, lamotrigine, or valproate (but monitor for metabolic syndrome).

Others

Pregabalin can cause significant weight gain but, similarly to valproate, does not seem to cause clinically significant changes in cholesterol[78] or increase the risk of MI[75]. Most studies examining these clinical outcomes are conducted in people with epilepsy, which itself may be a risk factor for cardiovascular events[79]. Where studies do control for the indication for the antiepileptic drug, however, the associations appear to remain[75].

The manufacturers of **promethazine** advise caution in patients with severe coronary artery disease, but the exact reason for this is not clear. As described above, promethazine may prolong the QT interval, but its torsadogenic potential is low[33]. Similarly, the use of **diphenhydramine** is cautioned by the manufacturers in cardiovascular disease, presumably due to effects on QT interval. Otherwise, antihistamines appear to be safe. **Benzodiazepines** are used in the management of acute coronary syndrome, and limited data suggest they improve cardiac mortality risk post MI when used in low or moderate doses[40]. This may be a result of better management of anxiety, rather than a direct effect of the drugs themselves. Higher doses have been associated with increased cardiac mortality[80].

As described above, the **cholinesterase inhibitors** may prolong the QT interval, so caution is advised in patients who are newly post MI. Otherwise, along with **memantine**, they may be protective for cardiovascular outcomes in coronary heart disease[81], possibly due to a reduction in myocardial revascularisation[43,82,83]. For older adults, particularly those at risk of a cardiac event, the importance of minimising the total anticholinergic burden of prescribed medication is becoming increasingly clear. A recent case-case-time-control study found an association between anticholinergic burden and acute cardiovascular events, with greater burdens conferring higher risk[84]. Use a tool such as Medichec (medichec.com) to calculate anticholinergic burden and deprescribe or select drugs with a lower score where possible.

HYPERTENSION

Depression and anxiety in hypertension

A relationship between hypertension and depression has been discussed since as early as 1898, when blood pressure was noted to rise in patients with depression[85]. Since then, research has suggested that the relationship may be bidirectional. Depression is an independent risk factor for developing hypertension[86], and the 'vascular depression' hypothesis proposes that cerebrovascular disease, for which hypertension is a risk factor, causes microvascular brain damage that may drive some depressive symptoms[87]. In contrast, studies in healthy populations show higher systolic blood pressure to be linked to a better mood and increased well-being[88]. Recently, a large UK imaging study with a 10-year follow-up time confirmed these two apparently contradictory associations – higher systolic blood pressure is linked to fewer depressive symptoms, and a diagnosis of hypertension is associated with more depressive symptoms[89]. The authors suggest that there may be a shared mechanism between subjective experience, emotional processing and pain that involves regulatory baroreceptors.

Anxiety was predictive of incidence of hypertension in the Framingham Heart Study[90], a finding also demonstrated in earlier studies[91] and confirmed in meta-analyses[92]. Further, patients with hypertension may be at heightened risk of developing anxiety, possibly a result of fear of the diagnosis[93]. It may be that sympathetic nervous system hyperactivity and cardiovascular oxidative stress contribute to the relationship[94].

Psychosis and bipolar disorder in hypertension

Meta-analysis suggests a prevalence for hypertension in schizophrenia of 39%[95], but rates may be higher in some areas (58% in the USA[48], 54% in England[96]). A higher risk of hypertension is also found in bipolar disorder[97,98], and in both conditions, treatment of hypertension is poor[98]. The presence of metabolic disorder is clearly important, and antipsychotics add to this risk. Other factors may also be influential; a genetic link between cardiometabolic disease and bipolar disorder is suggested[99], and inflammation and autonomic activity in psychosis may also be contributory[100].

Antidepressants

Hypertension and depression may share some pathology – both may involve overactivation of the sympathetic nervous system. Blockade of noradrenergic receptors in the heart, as well as centrally, may further sensitise the heart to sympathetic activation, increasing cardiac output and blood pressure[101]. This may be further exacerbated by drugs that block noradrenaline receptors, such as TCAs and SNRIs. Indeed, TCAs (and MAOIs) are associated with a risk of hypertensive crisis, and noradrenergic drugs (venlafaxine, duloxetine) are associated with dose-dependent increases in blood pressure[102] (although the effect for venlafaxine is not clinically significant at doses below 200mg/day, and even above this is only significant for about 5% of patients[103]). The anticholinergic effects of drugs such as TCAs may also contribute to increases in systolic blood pressure[102]. None is recommended for patients with pre-existing hypertension.

SSRIs do not appear to affect blood pressure[104] and are therefore preferable.

Recommendation: sertraline.

Antipsychotics

Antipsychotics may cause hypertension either acutely, via α_2 adrenergic receptor antagonism, or chronically, due to weight gain. Olanzapine, risperidone, and particularly clozapine have higher affinity for α_2-adrenergic receptors than other antipsychotics[12], making sharp rises in blood pressure on initiation of these drugs more likely, due to noradrenaline-mediated vasoconstriction. Olanzapine and clozapine are associated with more weight gain than other antipsychotics[24], which increases the risk of developing (or worsening) hypertension.

Recommendation: avoid olanzapine and risperidone.

Mood stabilisers

Hypertension has been rarely described in case reports with carbamazepine[105] and valproate[106,107], although causality is not certain. Lithium[108] and lamotrigine are not associated with hypertension.

Recommendation: all mood stabilisers are likely to be safe.

Others

Pregabalin and **promethazine**[109] are not associated with hypertension. The manufacturers of **diphenhydramine** caution against its use in hypertension when given parenterally, as large intravenous doses produce a strongly anticholinergic effect[110], but this does not appear to be a significant problem when taken orally. **Benzodiazepines** have hypotensive effects[111], possibly due to potentiation of the inhibitory effect of GABA and vasodilation[112]. Of the **anticholinesterase inhibitors**, rivastigmine has been rarely associated with hypertension in post-marketing surveillance, and hypertension is commonly reported as an adverse effect with galantamine. Donepezil does not appear to cause problems with blood pressure. Hypertension is common with **memantine** (4.1% of patients compared with 2.8% taking placebo[113]).

STROKE

Depression, anxiety, and stroke

Post-stroke depression is common, with a third of stroke survivors developing depression at some point after the event[114]. The frequency is highest in the first year, affecting one in three patients[115]. The South London Stroke Register found the cumulative incidence to be 55%[116], positioning post-stroke depression as the norm rather than the exception. Various reasons for this have been postulated, including (1) depression being a risk factor for stroke; (2) both depression and stroke having risk factors in common; (3) depression being a psychological reaction to stroke; (4) depression being secondary to other stroke outcomes, such as cognitive impairment; and (5) stroke having a direct pathophysiological effect on the brain[116]. Post-stroke mood disorders are strictly defined by the Diagnostic and Statistical Manual 5 (DSM-5) as mood disorders *due to* stroke, but the ability to definitively determine causality in clinical practice is lacking. Trials generally include symptoms of depression appearing at any time point post-stroke and include patients who had pre-existing depression diagnoses. The most consistent predictors of post-stroke depression are physical disability, stroke severity, a history of depression, and cognitive impairment[115]. It is associated with poorer functional outcomes after stroke[115].

Anxiety is also common post-stroke, with about one in four patients affected[117]. Comorbid depression is common[118]. Evidence to support optimal treatment choice is sparse[119], despite an association of severe post-stroke anxiety with poor outcomes and quality of life[120].

Psychosis, bipolar disorder, and stroke

Schizophrenia[8,121] and bipolar disorder[8,122,123] are associated with an increased risk of stroke, with SMI as a whole conferring a two-fold increased risk[122]. This is likely to be a result of the increased cardiovascular comorbidity in SMI, including diabetes, hypertension, and hyperlipidaemia. Not only is there an increased likelihood of stroke but there is also increased mortality post-stroke in both the short (30-day) and long (5-year) term[122,124]. This may be a consequence suboptimal clinical care. Studies done in various countries worldwide have shown that patients with schizophrenia are less likely to receive thrombolysis or carotid imaging, be screened for hyperlipidaemia, be prescribed antihypertensives or anticoagulants, achieve target lipid levels post-stroke, or receive outpatient stroke care[125-129]. In one study, this translated to mortality at 1-year post-stroke in patients over 70 years of 47%, compared with 35% for those without schizophrenia[126].

Antidepressants

SSRIs and nortriptyline are widely recommended as the antidepressants of choice post-stroke[12]. They may be associated with less dependence on carers post-stroke, less disability, less neurological impairment, and less anxiety and depression, including in people without a diagnosis of depression[130]. Treatment with fluoxetine or nortriptyline has been shown to reduce long-term mortality in comparison with placebo, including in patients who were not depressed at baseline[131]. This protective effect appears to remain even if antidepressants are only given for a short period following the stroke, suggesting that the mortality risk exceeds the duration of the depression[131]. SSRIs, however, are problematic to use in patients also taking anticoagulants (inevitable if the stroke was ischaemic) or at risk of bleeding for other reasons (those who suffered haemorrhagic stroke). Nortriptyline is more attractive in this regard. Mirtazapine and agomelatine largely avoid issues with bleeding, but data supporting use post-stroke are entirely lacking for agomelatine and are conflicting for mirtazapine. One cohort study suggested an increased risk of a second stroke with mirtazapine, although this was in older adults, and the risk appears to reduce with time. This may reflect the fact that undertreated depression itself is a risk factor for stroke[132]. Other studies support the safety and efficacy of mirtazapine post-stroke[133,134].

Recommendation: nortriptyline or mirtazapine if bleeding is a concern, but monitor for weight gain with mirtazapine. Otherwise, SSRI.

Antipsychotics

The association of antipsychotics with a heightened risk of stroke in elderly patients with dementia is well described. What this means for younger patients without dementia, who are taking antipsychotics for other mental illnesses, is less clear. Few studies specifically address this question, and where they do exist they use heterogeneous outcomes (stroke incidence versus mortality from stroke, for example) and durations of follow-up (weeks to years). The impact of changes in antipsychotic prescription type is not clearly accounted for, and confounding by indication is difficult to control. Where studies attempt to report risk of stroke by drug type, this is usually by 'first-generation' versus 'second-generation' drugs, and results are conflicting.

Some studies report different results depending on stroke type (one Taiwanese study found an increased risk of ischaemic stroke, but not haemorrhagic, with atypical drugs)[135]; others do not report the stroke subtypes separately[136]. Systematic review and meta-analyses also draw different conclusions depending on their chosen inclusion criteria[67,136]. Overall, it seems possible that antipsychotics may increase the risk of stroke. Whether this is due to some direct, acutely mediated effect is not clear. It is certainly the case that antipsychotics increase the risk of obesity and insulin resistance, which in turn are risk factors for cardiovascular and cerebrovascular disease. They are also associated with an increased risk of venous thromboembolism. At the moment, there are insufficient data to support choosing one drug over another, but minimising weight gain is important.

Recommendation: no obvious optimal choice. Avoid weight gain.

Mood stabilisers

Animal models show a neuroprotective effect of lithium post-stroke[137], and a few small trials suggest this benefit may translate into humans[138], although data are as yet very limited[139]. In terms of *de novo* stroke, lithium appears to confer either no extra risk[140], or possibly a reduced risk[141]. Variation in the histone deacetylase 9 gene (HDAC9) has been identified as a cause of large artery stroke. Inhibiting the activity of the HDAC9 protein might therefore reduce the risk of stroke, and one drug that has this activity is sodium valproate. Data so far available suggest that this might be the case[77,142] (but note one case-crossover study finding an increased risk of haemorrhagic stroke with acute use of valproate in bipolar disorder[140]). Lamotrigine appears to be safe[140,143]. Carbamazepine is associated with a higher risk of stroke than the other mood-stabilising antiepileptics[77,140] and should be avoided.

Recommendation: lithium, valproate, lamotrigine.

Others

Pregabalin is widely used in the treatment of pain post-stroke[144], and as with lithium, animal studies suggest a role in brain recovery[145]. Similarly, **promethazine** may be anti-inflammatory post-stroke[146]. **Diphenhydramine** is not known to pose a problem in stroke.

Animal models show a neuroprotective effect for GABA receptor agonists such as **benzodiazepines** in cerebrovascular disease, but this does not appear to extend to improvement in outcomes for acute stroke in people[147]. Benzodiazepine use may in fact increase mortality post-stroke[148], and there may be a dose-related increased risk of incident stroke[149]. This may be due in part to an increased risk of pneumonia for patients taking benzodiazepines[150], oversedation increasing the need for intubation, or higher incidence of falls. However, there are many confounding factors, including the increased likelihood of benzodiazepine use, particularly in patients who have other predictors of mortality such as delirium, agitation, or anxiety post-stroke, and so a direct causal association has been disputed[151]. Nonetheless, it is prudent to avoid use where possible and to minimise doses where not possible.

Acetylcholinesterase inhibitors may be protective for ischaemic stroke, possibly because of a protective effect on endothelial cells and anti-inflammatory mediated reduction in atherosclerosis[152]. They may also improve cognitive and functional impairment post-stroke[153,154]. **Memantine** may exert similar neuroprotective effects from stroke by inhibition of NMDA channels, reducing excitotoxic injury[155]. Not all studies examining the safety of acetylcholinesterase inhibitors control for concurrent use of antipsychotics, which are known to increase the risk of stroke in dementia. Other confounders are also important, including BMI and physical activity, hypertension, and smoking. These discrepancies in study design may explain the findings by some of an increased stroke risk in previous users of acetylcholinesterase inhibitors[156]. However, the consensus is that they, and memantine, are likely to be safe.

ATRIAL FIBRILLATION

Depression, anxiety, and atrial fibrillation

Depression increases the risk of developing atrial fibrillation[157,158], and the prevalence of depression is higher in patients with atrial fibrillation than in the general population (8–38% vs 1–2%)[157]. The reasons for this may be similar to those for other cardiac conditions, including inflammation, oxidative stress, autonomic nerve function, hypothalamic-pituitary-adrenal axis imbalance, and the burden of cardiac symptoms on quality of life[159]. This association extends to an increased risk of recurrence of atrial fibrillation after catheter ablation in patients with depression[160]. As with other cardiac conditions, depression is also associated with increased cardiovascular mortality in atrial fibrillation[161]. Depression and atrial fibrillation are both associated with non-adherence to cardiac treatment regimens[162], and this may contribute to the increase in mortality risk[163].

Chronic stress and anxiety may increase the risk of atrial fibrillation in the same way as for depression, through inflammation, oxidative stress, and increased sympathetic activity resulting in catecholamine overload[164]. Anxiety is a risk factor for mortality in patients with coronary heart disease and atrial fibrillation[165].

Psychosis, bipolar disorder, and atrial fibrillation

Patients with schizophrenia and bipolar disorder have a higher likelihood of developing atrial fibrillation, with one study finding a two-fold higher risk[166]. Data are emerging to suggest a possible genetic link with schizophrenia[167]. Schizophrenia is associated with a poorer prognosis in atrial fibrillation, and Danish authors have shown that this may be linked to disparities in the quality of care for the cardiac condition. Patients with mental health conditions – including depression, bipolar disorder, anxiety, and schizophrenia – are less likely to receive antiarrhythmic therapy[168] or oral anticoagulation[163,169,170], and less likely to adhere to anticoagulation in the long term[171].

Risk factors for cardiovascular disease and mortality are common in serious mental illness and also play a part in the increased risk for ischaemic stroke, thromboembolic events, and major bleeding in patients with schizophrenia or bipolar disorder and atrial fibrillation[172].

Antidepressants

Serotonin promotes intracellular calcium overload, which is potentially arrhythmogenic[173]. Preclinical and clinical data show that stimulation of 5-HT_4 receptors can trigger sinus tachycardia and atrial arrhythmias[174]. Whether serotonergic antidepressants increase the risk of incident atrial fibrillation in practice is not entirely clear in the published literature. Given the known impact of depression on the risk of atrial fibrillation, there is a clear potential for confounding by indication, which is not always accounted for in meta-analyses on the subject[175]. This is demonstrated by a large Danish study, which found a three-fold higher risk of atrial fibrillation immediately before and after starting antidepressants, but the association gradually attenuated over the following year[176]. This suggests that treatment of depression may reduce the longer-term risk of developing atrial fibrillation. Other studies also find that antidepressants are not associated with atrial fibrillation[173], but some cast doubt on this conclusion[177,178]. More studies are needed that are specifically designed to look at whether possible proarrhythmic properties of antidepressants oppose the antiarrhythmic benefits of improving depressive symptoms.

TCAs should be avoided in patients with cardiac disease, as discussed earlier in this chapter. Their effects on slowing of intraventricular conduction mean that they are generally contraindicated in disorders of cardiac rhythm[179]. Mirtazapine and agomelatine appear to be safe choices in relation to cardiac conduction.

Other than an effect on the risk of atrial fibrillation itself, the obvious problem with antidepressants is that of bleeding risk. Stasis of blood in the atria during fibrillation predisposes to clot formation and substantially increases the risk of stroke, so anticoagulation is essential. See section on anticoagulation for more detail surrounding drug choice.

The ideal choice of antidepressant in atrial fibrillation is therefore one that strikes a favourable balance between risk to cardiac conduction and risk of additive bleeding with concurrent anticoagulants. Mirtazapine and agomelatine are the least likely to cause problems in either regard (although mirtazapine is not entirely without bleeding risk; see anticoagulation section). TCAs are less likely to cause bleeding problems than SSRIs but are probably less safe in cardiac disease.

Recommendation: mirtazapine or agomelatine. SSRIs can be used, but beware of the interaction with warfarin and other anticoagulants.

Antipsychotics

Atrial fibrillation is described in case reports to be associated with aripiprazole[180,181], clozapine[182,183], olanzapine[182,184] and paliperidone[185], and a nested case control study found current antipsychotic use to be associated with a 17% increased risk of atrial fibrillation relative to non-users[186]. The reason for this apparent association is not clear, but cardiovascular comorbidities such as hypertension, diabetes, and coronary heart disease are very likely play a part. Other proposed mechanisms include effects on the autonomic nervous system, cardiac muscarinic blockage[186], and stimulation of the hypothalamic-pituitary-adrenal axis[187]. There is evidence that compared with controls, patients with schizophrenia are more likely to have an increased heart rate, QTc prolongation, and pathological Q waves. In one study, patients taking any antipsychotic, especially clozapine or multiple concurrent antipsychotics, were particularly likely to have an abnormal ECG (predominantly QTc prolongation, right or left conduction disturbances, or pathological Q waves)[188]. Aripiprazole was the only antipsychotic not implicated in this effect. Interestingly, this study found no association between atrial fibrillation and antipsychotics (or schizophrenia).

Recommendation: cariprazine, brexpiprazole, lurasidone, lumateperone. Aripiprazole may also be used but is not entirely without effect on the QT interval.

Mood stabilisers

Valproate does not appear to be associated with atrial fibrillation, other than a single case report of atrioventricular conduction block[189]. Carbamazepine and lamotrigine are not associated with atrial fibrillation. Lithium also seems safe but ECG changes, including atrial fibrillation, are known to occur in acute and chronic intoxication[190]. Ensuring plasma concentrations are kept within therapeutic ranges is therefore even more important in a patient with pre-existing atrial fibrillation.

Recommendation: all options are safe.

Others

Two case reports implicate **pregabalin** in the development of atrial fibrillation, although both were patients hospitalised for infections[191,192]. One study in elderly patients found a dose-related increased incidence of initiation of antiarrhythmic drugs and anticoagulants in patients in the 3 months after starting pregabalin (or gabapentin)[193]. This finding has yet to be replicated but should perhaps prompt extra caution (cardiac monitoring for 3 months) in elderly patients.

Promethazine was associated with a higher risk of hospitalisation for atrial fibrillation in elderly patients than loratadine or betahistine in one study conducted in Denmark[194]. The risk was higher in patients with prior cardiac arrhythmias, heart failure, or those on other arrhythmogenic drugs. The authors postulate that this may be due to prolongation of the QT interval, which is known to predispose to atrial fibrillation[195]. As discussed earlier in this chapter, other authors have found that although promethazine is associated with QT interval prolongation, it is at a subclinical level that is not torsadogenic[33]. Of note, the Danish study found no association between promethazine use and myocardial infarction. The authors hypothesise that the association between promethazine and atrial fibrillation in their study was the result of subclinical QT interval prolongation adding arrhythmogenic potential to patients already at risk due to their age and history of cardiac disease.

There are no other published reports of an association between promethazine and atrial fibrillation and given the widespread use of the drug it seems likely that at most, this must be a rare event. Promethazine (and other anticholinergic drugs) should be avoided where possible in elderly patients due to negative effects on cognition, sedation, and falls[196]. The dramatic increase in risk of atrial fibrillation found in this study adds to these concerns, particularly in elderly patients with a history of cardiac disease, but requires replication. **Diphenhydramine** is not associated with atrial fibrillation.

A recent, large Taiwanese cohort study found an increased incidence of atrial fibrillation in patients taking hypnotics, including **benzodiazepines**[197]. The effect was dose-related. The reason for this association may be confounding by indication (hypnotics are more likely to be prescribed to people with psychiatric disorders, which themselves are risk factors for atrial fibrillation), or observation bias (people taking hypnotics are more likely to visit a clinician and have a routine ECG that then identifies asymptomatic atrial fibrillation). A further possibility is a direct effect of GABA-mediated inhibition of the sympathetic and parasympathetic nervous system having a detrimental effect on cardiac autonomic function. Whatever the cause of the association, it is clearly wise to minimise the use of benzodiazepines in all patients, including those with cardiac disease. There is also an increased risk of falls in elderly patients with atrial fibrillation[198], which is increased further in patients who take benzodiazepines[199].

The **acetylcholinesterase inhibitors** are known to cause bradycardia, which may be problematic in patients with supraventricular cardiac conduction conditions such as paroxysmal atrial fibrillation. Otherwise, ECG changes or arrhythmias are rare[200,201]. Donepezil may be more associated with QT prolongation than rivastigmine or galantamine, but the evidence for this is inconclusive and limited to case reports, and the potential mechanism for any differences between the drugs is unclear[201]. **Memantine** is not associated with cardiac arrhythmia. Preclinical models suggest it may even be able to prevent and terminate atrial fibrillation[202].

ANTICOAGULATION

Antidepressants

Serotonergic antidepressants are associated with an increased risk of bleeding and of a prolonged duration or severity of bleeding (not restricted to gastrointestinal bleeds) and this is likely to be related to the affinity of the drug for the serotonin transporter on platelets. Drugs that have weak (or no) affinity for the serotonin transporter are preferred for patients at risk of bleeding, including those taking concurrent anticoagulants (warfarin or non-vitamin K antagonists), who are at increased risk of bleeding if also given a serotonergic antidepressant[203,204].

Options include trazodone, mianserin, reboxetine, dosulepin, moclobemide, nortriptyline, phenelzine, trimipramine, lofepramine, mirtazapine and agomelatine. Trazodone and mianserin are recommended by the UK National Institute for Health and Care Excellence (NICE)[13], but trazodone may increase digoxin levels[205]. Reboxetine is not effective and there is a risk of hypokalaemia and hypocalcaemia when it is given with diuretics[205]. TCAs are proarrhythmic and TCAs and MAOIs are associated with increased blood pressure. Mirtazapine and agomelatine are probably safer alternatives, although note the risk of weight gain with mirtazapine. A small study in healthy subjects showed a minor increase in the INR when mirtazapine was combined with warfarin[206] (the mean increased from 1.6 to 1.8). This was not considered clinically significant, but two case reports describe much larger increases in INR[207,208]. Monitor INR if mirtazapine is added to warfarin, at initiation and at dose changes. There is also evidence of an increased bleeding risk when mirtazapine is combined with non-vitamin K antagonist oral anticoagulants (NOACs)[209].

Recommendation: mirtazapine or agomelatine.

Antipsychotics

Analogous to serotonergic antidepressants, antipsychotics that are antagonists at the 5-HT_{2A} receptor may also affect platelet aggregation, and therefore theoretically contribute to an increased risk of prolonged bleeding. A single case-control study suggested an increased risk of gastrointestinal and intracranial bleeding for patients taking antipsychotics[210], but did not find an association between the degree of affinity with the 5-HT_{2A} receptor, and has yet to be replicated.

There is a further issue to consider where patients are taking NOACs. NOACs are substrates of P-glycoprotein, metabolised by CYP3A4. Antipsychotics that are CYP3A4 and/or P-glycoprotein inhibitors may therefore increase the plasma concentration of NOACs, enhancing their anticoagulant effect and increasing the risk of prolonged bleeding. Drugs such as haloperidol and quetiapine, which are mainly metabolised by CYP3A4 and also inhibit P-glycoprotein, may be more likely to cause major bleeding events than antipsychotics such as olanzapine, where CYP3A4 plays a more minor role in metabolism[211]. However, specific evidence for an interaction effect between antipsychotics and NOACs is limited. Pharmacokinetic studies that examine NOAC plasma concentrations in combination with other drugs show that significant interaction effects occur mainly with substances that strongly inhibit both the CYP3A4 and P-glycoprotein pathways. The clinical effect for antipsychotics is therefore likely to be minimal. One large Taiwanese cohort study found an increased risk of bleeding when patients with atrial fibrillation were exposed to a NOAC and an antipsychotic, with the highest risk seen in patients taking haloperidol[211].

When using antipsychotics for behavioural symptoms in dementia or delirium in elderly patients, and especially if there is concurrent renal impairment (which also increases NOAC plasma concentrations), consider avoiding haloperidol and quetiapine and choose olanzapine or aripiprazole (drugs less associated with a higher risk of bleeding in the cohort study). Otherwise, there is currently no evidence to strongly support changing standard practice.

In contrast to the foregoing, antipsychotics are also associated with an increased risk of venous thromboembolism, particularly at the start of treatment[212]. This may be relevant if considering treatment options in patients who have already experienced a thromboembolic event and may be at risk of another, and particularly if antipsychotics are not definitively indicated in such patients (that is, another drug or non-drug measure could be used). The absolute risk is small – in a large, UK-based case-control study, there were an extra four cases of venous thromboembolism per 10,000 patients treated over 1 year across all age groups, and 10 for patients aged 65 and over[212].

Recommendation: all antipsychotics are associated with a small risk of thromboembolism. Avoid haloperidol and quetiapine in patients taking NOACs.

Mood stabilisers

Sodium valproate causes a variety of haematological abnormalities, including inhibition of platelet aggregation and thrombocytopenia[213], but the clinical significance of this is disputed. Some retrospective studies demonstrate an increase in perioperative bleeding, others do not[214]. Most of the published data are in children undergoing neurosurgery for epilepsy. How this should be interpreted for adults taking valproate for mental health disorders is unclear – children appear to be more at risk of valproate-induced coagulopathies than adults[215]. Retrospective studies have found an association between heavy menstrual bleeding and valproate in women with serious mental illness[216]. Descriptions of severe (or even fatal) haemorrhage in adult patients are limited to case reports (again, in epilepsy)[217-219]. Thrombocytopenia and bleeding are reported at both supratherapeutic and subtherapeutic plasma concentrations. Valproate is an inducer of CYP3A4 and P-glycoprotein, which may result in lower plasma concentrations of NOACs. This has led to the combination being contraindicated by the European Society of Cardiology[220], although evidence of the interaction in clinical practice is limited[221,222].

Carbamazepine is a potent CYP3A4 and P-glycoprotein inducer, and therefore increases the metabolism of both vitamin K antagonists and NOACs. This is clinically important, resulting in increased incidence of thrombotic events[223,224]. Consider also the risk of overcoagulation if carbamazepine is stopped in a patient taking an anticoagulant, if doses have been adjusted during co-treatment to account for the interaction. Lamotrigine does not interact with anticoagulants or increase the risk of bleeding. Lithium is also free of anticoagulant drug interactions, and not associated with an increased risk of bleeding (in fact, preclinical studies suggest it may be neuroprotective after intracranial haemorrhage[225]).

Recommendation: lithium, lamotrigine.

Others

As for lithium, **pregabalin** does not interact with anticoagulants, is not associated with an increased risk of bleeding, and is suggested in preclinical studies to be neuroprotective after intracranial haemorrhage[226]. **Promethazine, diphenhydramine,** and **benzodiazepines** are not known to cause problems with bleeding or anticoagulation.

Case reports have suggested a link between **acetylcholinesterase inhibitors** and bleeding events[227–229]. This may be due to inhibition of platelet activation, as acetylcholine is thought to be an endogenous inhibitor of platelets[230]. Limited data from cohort and case-control studies do not seem to support this theory, with several studies failing to find an association with bleeding events and acetylcholinesterase inhibitors[156,231]. **Memantine** is not associated with an increased risk of bleeds.

ADHD MEDICATION IN ADULTS WITH CARDIAC DISEASE

The stimulant drugs methylphenidate and dexamphetamine, and the non-stimulant atomoxetine, carry manufacturers' warnings contraindicating use in a range of cardiovascular disorders. These warnings include severe hypertension, heart failure, arterial occlusive disease, angina, congenital heart disease, cardiomyopathy, myocardial infarction, life-threatening arrhythmias, and channelopathies. Cerebrovascular disorders, including cerebral aneurysms, vasculitis, and stroke, also contraindicate use. Lisdexamphetamine, the prodrug of dexamphetamine, is contraindicated in symptomatic cardiovascular disease and moderate hypertension.

These contraindications arose from two observations: post-marketing surveillance reports of sudden death, stroke and myocardial infarction in adults taking CNS stimulant treatments; and sudden deaths in paediatric patients with structural cardiac abnormalities taking stimulants for ADHD[232,233]. In response to these naturalistic observations, two large retrospective cohort studies were conducted. The first included more than a million children and young adults, examined ADHD medicines (including methylphenidate, dexamphetamine, and atomoxetine), and failed to find any evidence of an increased risk of serious cardiovascular events[234]. The second examined over half a million participants between the ages of 25 and 64, and also failed to find any association between ADHD medication and an increased risk of cardiovascular events[235].

Since then, other studies have produced conflicting results. For example, a case-only study conducted in over a thousand children in South Korea found an increased risk of arrhythmia and myocardial infarction[236]. Differences in study design may account for the varying results reported in the literature, reflecting the difficulty in studying an outcome that is extremely rare, particularly in children. Adults with ADHD are likely to have more risk factors for cardiovascular or cerebrovascular adverse events than children, being more likely to smoke, be obese, and take other medicines, as well as already having cardiac disease. ADHD itself may be an independent risk factor for developing cardiovascular disease[237]. Cohort studies in adults taking ADHD medication produce inconsistent results, some finding no increased risk of cardiovascular events (myocardial infarction or stroke) for any ADHD medication[235]. In contrast, a large cohort study in adults found an increased risk of ventricular arrhythmia in people taking methylphenidate, but the dose was inversely associated with risk, suggesting the association may not be causal[238]. Another cohort study found an increased risk of transient ischaemic attack in adult users of atomoxetine, but no increased risk of stroke[239].

Recent meta-analysis suggests overall no increased risk of cardiovascular disease with ADHD medication in adults or children (methylphenidate, amphetamines, and atomoxetine)[240], including in those with pre-existing cardiovascular disease, although the authors noted that more data are required and an increased risk of myocardial infarction or tachyarrhythmia could not be excluded. Lisdexamphetamine is comparatively less studied, but as a pro-drug of dexamphetamine has a similar safety profile to the other stimulants[241]. A cohort study in adult patients concluded that there was little or no increased risk of cardiovascular or cerebrovascular events in patients taking lisdexamphetamine, compared with those previously treated with other ADHD medication[242].

Older adults have an increased baseline risk for cardiovascular events, as well as being more likely to take several other drugs, increasing the likelihood of drug interactions and additive adverse effects. Fewer data are available for this population, and as for other age groups, published studies draw conflicting conclusions. One cohort study of stimulants in adults over 66 years found an increased risk of cardiac events (in particular, ventricular arrhythmia, stroke, or transient ischaemic attack) in the first 30 days of treatment[243], but the risk attenuated over time, with no association with cardiac adverse events at 6 or 12 months. Other studies that included older adults did not find any relationship with cardiac events[244], and a meta-analysis overall found no statistically significant association[240].

There is biological plausibility for an association with ADHD medicines and cardiovascular adverse events. The stimulants and atomoxetine are known to cause small rises in blood pressure and heart rate (they are sympathomimetic agents)[245,246]. Average blood pressure increases reported in studies are small (3 to 6mmHg systolic, 2 to 4mmHg diastolic), and some degree of tolerance may develop over time[247]. Average reported heart rate increases are 4 to 5bpm[247]. The stimulants and atomoxetine[247] are also proarrhythmogenic because of beta-adrenergic stimulation of the heart[248], potentially worsening atrial fibrillation or tachycardias, but it is not clear whether this translates into a direct association with adverse cardiac outcomes, as the previously described observational studies demonstrate. These drugs have also been shown to reduce heart rate variability and increase arterial stiffness[249]. Other sympathomimetic drugs have also been associated with adverse cardiac outcomes[250].

Summary

The absolute contraindication of these medicines in cardiovascular disease is not cogently supported by current evidence[247]. Serious cardiac or cerebrovascular events in patients taking ADHD medicines are rare, and their risk may be outweighed by the benefits of the medication. Patients with pre-existing cardiovascular disease have a higher baseline risk of a further adverse event before adding to this risk with ADHD medication, and this should be considered when weighing against the potential benefits.

Recommendations

- Be aware of the medicolegal implications of prescribing in context of a manufacturer's contraindication.
- Where possible, avoid the use of stimulants or atomoxetine in patients with cardiovascular or cerebrovascular disease. Use non-drug options or other medication in preference.
- Blood pressure and heart rate increases are not usually clinically significant. Some tolerance to the effects of the medicines on these parameters may develop over time. Do not stop the medication unless it is clinically necessary to do so.
- Patients with proarrhythmic cardiovascular diseases may be at particular risk from stimulants and atomoxetine. These drugs should only be used in this group of patients if there is clear benefit, and after other treatment options have been exhausted.
- The stimulant drugs and atomoxetine do not usually cause any apparent ECG changes. Therefore, ECG monitoring is probably of limited value in predicting a patient's risk of developing a drug-induced arrhythmia, or experiencing sudden cardiac death[247]. Nonetheless, a baseline ECG is recommended. The need for ongoing ECG monitoring should be discussed with a cardiologist.

DRUG–DRUG INTERACTIONS[205,251,252]

There is a theoretical risk of additive hypotension when any antipsychotic or tricyclic antidepressant is given alongside an antihypertensive medicine.

ACE inhibitors

ACE inhibitors can cause SIADH and resultant hyponatraemia. All antidepressants and antipsychotics, and carbamazepine, have been associated with the development of hyponatraemia – the risk is highest in the first weeks of treatment[21]. Monitor sodium levels in the first month of treatment, especially in patients with other risk factors for developing hyponatraemia.

The interaction between lithium and ACE inhibitors is well known. ACE inhibitors can cause dehydration (due to reduction in thirst), which can increase lithium plasma concentrations. They also increase renal sodium loss, which in turn also increases lithium plasma concentrations. The magnitude of the effect is unpredictable. Some patients are unaffected, others experience four-fold increases in lithium levels[12]. If the combination is unavoidable, monitor lithium plasma concentrations and renal function closely (weekly until stable, then at least 3 monthly).

Angiotensin-II antagonists

There are case reports of lithium toxicity when given with the angiotensin-II antagonists candesartan, losartan, valsartan, and irbesartan. Similar to the ACE inhibitors, the angiotensin-II inhibitors inhibit aldosterone secretion in the kidneys, resulting in increased sodium loss by the renal tubules. This causes lithium retention and a risk of toxicity. The effect is not as marked as it is for ACE inhibitors, and evidence in clinical use is limited to a few case reports. As for ACE inhibitors, monitor lithium plasma concentrations weekly until stable (which may take up to eight weeks).

Beta blockers

Sotalol has a high risk of prolonging the QT interval. Combination with antidepressants, especially TCAs, citalopram, and escitalopram, should be avoided. Similarly, avoid the combination of sotalol with antipsychotics that prolong the QT interval, or lithium. Duloxetine, fluoxetine, and paroxetine (and to a lesser extent, citalopram and escitalopram) inhibit CYP2D6, and so may increase exposure to propranolol, metoprolol, carvedilol, and nebivolol.

Calcium channel blockers

The non-dihydropyridine calcium channel blockers diltiazem and verapamil are moderate inhibitors of CYP3A4. There is therefore a theoretical risk of an increased plasma concentration of drugs such as trazodone, vilazodone, cariprazine, lurasidone, lumateperone, brexpiprazole, iloperidone, risperidone, paliperidone, quetiapine, droperidol, sertindole, and pimozide.

Concurrent use of cariprazine and CYP3A4 inhibitors is contraindicated by the UK manufacturers. The FDA allows prescribing with strong CYP3A4 inhibitors, with dose adjustment of cariprazine. It recommends reducing the dose by half, or to alternate days for patients taking 1.5mg. New starters of cariprazine should be started at 1.5mg on day 1 and 3 (no dose on day 2), then 1.5mg daily, up to a maximum of 3mg. Lumateperone doses should be reduced to 21mg daily if given with diltiazem or verapamil, and lurasidone doses should be halved. Brexpiprazole doses should be reduced if a concurrent CYP2D6 inhibitor is also given. The UK manufacturers of sertindole contraindicate diltazem and verapamil, principally because if a patient is also a poor metaboliser of CYP2D6, the CYP3A4 pathway becomes more important. This seems overcautious. In the UK, quetiapine is contraindicated with all CYP3A4 inhibitors, based on evidence of increased plasma concentrations with strong inhibitors such as ketoconazole. Advice is more nuanced in the USA, where dose reductions to one sixth of the original dose are recommended only with strong inhibitors.

TCAs are predominantly metabolised via CYP2D6, but 3A4 is a minor pathway. This may explain observations in a few case reports and one crossover study of increased plasma concentrations of trimipramine, nortriptyline and imipramine when combined with verapamil, and in particular diltiazem. The crossover study[253] (conducted in 12 healthy males, ethnicity not reported) showed an increase in plasma concentrations of a single dose of imipramine of 15% when given with verapamil, and 30% when given with diltiazem. Two of the participants developed second-degree heart block on the combination of imipramine and verapamil. A mean PR interval of >200ms was observed in both diltiazem and verapamil groups, representing first-degree heart block. Beyond this study, there is scant evidence for a clinically significant interaction between calcium channel blockers and TCAs. The combination is not contraindicated, or even cautioned by manufacturers. TCAs should be avoided in patients with significant cardiac disease, but if they are to be used in combination with diltiazem or verapamil in a patient at particular risk of heart block, monitor the ECG and dose cautiously.

Carbamazepine reduces the concentration of calcium channel blockers (it is a potent CYP3A4 inducer). Conversely, carbamazepine is also metabolised by CYP3A4, and so the moderate inhibitors diltiazem and verapamil may increase carbamazepine concentrations. Use plasma concentrations to guide dosing. There are some reports of neurotoxicity and alterations in lithium plasma concentrations when lithium is given with calcium channel blockers, but also reports of uneventful use. The mechanism for a potential interaction is unclear.

Sacubitril/valsartan

No interactions, but note that the manufacturer mentions hallucinations, paranoia, and sleep disturbance (in the context of psychotic events). The cautions described for angiotensin-II inhibitors also apply here.

Spironolactone/eplerenone

The manufacturer of eplerenone cautions against the combination with lithium, apparently because of the risk of lithium toxicity with diuretics and ACE inhibitors. There is no clear evidence of a serious interaction between lithium and potassium-sparing diuretics, but measuring lithium plasma levels on initiation would be wise. There is also a manufacturer's warning of the risk of hypotension with all 'neuroleptics' (antipsychotics), and tricyclic antidepressants when combined with eplerenone. Exposure to eplerenone may be reduced by the CYP3A4 inducer carbamazepine.

Ivabradine

Ivabradine causes bradycardia, which increases the risk of torsade de pointes in people with a prolonged QTc – caution should be exercised when combining with antidepressants or antipsychotics that prolong the QT, or lithium. Due to CYP3A4 induction, carbamazepine may reduce the plasma concentration of ivabradine.

Digoxin

Isolated case reports and a single case-control study suggest the possibility of increased plasma levels of digoxin with fluoxetine, fluvoxamine, paroxetine or sertraline[254], but this is disputed. Clinically significant problems are highly unlikely.

Hydralazine

The manufacturer notes a risk of enhanced hypotensive effect when hydralazine is combined with TCAs or clozapine.

Nitrates

Nitrates are known to cause postural hypotension, particularly if combined with alcohol – TCAs, MAOIs, trazodone, and antipsychotics may add to this risk. The antimuscarinic effects of TCAs may cause dry mouth, which might affect the dissolution of glyceryl trinitrate sublingual tablets. Switching to a glyceryl trinitrate spray is a possible alternative.

Loop diuretics

Symptomatic hypotension caused by loop diuretics may be worsened by other drugs that cause hypotension (TCAs, MAOIs, trazodone, antipsychotics).

There is a possible increased risk of hypokalaemia when loop diuretics are given with reboxetine. Additionally, loop diuretics are known to cause hypokalaemia, and this increases the risk of torsade de pointes. Caution is advised if this occurs when combining with drugs known to prolong the QT interval (TCAs, citalopram, escitalopram, antipsychotics, lithium).

Patients taking diuretics may be at increased risk of developing hyponatraemia. This risk may be enhanced by concurrent use of other drugs that can cause hyponatraemia, including antidepressants, antipsychotics, and carbamazepine. Monitoring of sodium is advised, especially in the first 4 weeks of treatment and in patients with additional risk factors for hyponatraemia.

The manufacturers of risperidone advise particular caution when combining it with furosemide in elderly patients with dementia. This is because of a finding in two placebo-controlled studies of an increase in mortality with the combination. The reason for this is not clear (thiazide diuretics do not appear to have this association), but dehydration is a known risk factor for mortality. The use of the two drugs together is not contraindicated, but in practice if alternatives can be used, this would seem sensible.

Loop diuretics can cause increases in lithium plasma concentrations, possibly because of increased sodium loss and resorption. Many patients experience no difficulties with the combination, but there are reports of serious lithium toxicity. Monitor lithium plasma concentrations more frequently (ideally weekly) for the first month when starting the combination.

SUMMARY OF RECOMMENDATIONS

	Antidepressant	Antipsychotic	Mood stabiliser
Heart failure	Sertraline. Avoid TCAs.	Cariprazine, brexpiprazole, lumateperone or lurasidone. Avoid olanzapine. Note that clozapine may not be contraindicated.	No obvious optimal choice; see text.
Coronary heart disease	Sertraline, or mirtazapine if significant bleeding risk.	Cariprazine, brexpiprazole, lumateperone or lurasidone.	Lithium, lamotrigine. If using valproate or pregabalin monitor weight. Avoid carbamazepine.
Hypertension	Sertraline	Any, but avoid olanzapine and possibly risperidone.	Any
Anticoagulation	Mirtazapine, agomelatine	Any	Lithium, lamotrigine, pregabalin. Avoid carbamazepine and possibly valproate.
Stroke	Mirtazapine	No obvious optimal choice, see text. Avoid weight gain.	Lithium, valproate, lamotrigine, pregabalin. Avoid carbamazepine.
Atrial fibrillation	Mirtazapine or agomelatine. SSRIs can be used, but beware of the interaction with warfarin and other anticoagulants.	Cariprazine, brexpiprazole, lumateperone, or lurasidone.	Any

References

1. DiMatteo, M. R. *et al.* Depression is a risk factor for noncompliance with medical treatment meta-analysis of the effects of anxiety and depression on patient adherence. *Arch Int Med* 2000; **160**: 2101–2107, doi:10.1001/archinte.160.14.2101.

2. Celano, C. M. *et al.* Depression and anxiety in heart failure: a review. *Harv Rev Psychiatry* 2018; **26**(4): 175–184.

3. Celano, C. M. *et al.* Association between anxiety and mortality in patients with coronary artery disease: A meta-analysis. *Am Heart J* 2015; **170**: 1105–1115, doi:10.1016/j.ahj.2015.09.013.

4. Alhurani, A. S. *et al.* The association of co-morbid symptoms of depression and anxiety with all-cause mortality and cardiac rehospitalization in patients with heart failure. *Psychosomatics* 2015; **56**: 371–380, doi:10.1016/j.psym.2014.05.022.

5. O'Connor, C. M. *et al.* Safety and efficacy of sertraline for depression in patients with heart failure: Results of the SADHART-CHF (Sertraline against depression and heart disease in chronic heart failure) trial. *J Am Coll Cardiology* 2010; **56**: 692–699, doi:10.1016/j.jacc.2010.03.068.

6. Angermann, C. E. *et al.* Effect of escitalopram on all-cause mortality and hospitalization in patients with heart failure and depression the mood-hf randomized clinical trial. *JAMA* 2016; **315**, doi:10.1001/jama.2016.7635.

7. Nielsen, R. E. *et al.* Cardiovascular disease in patients with severe mental illness. *Nat Rev Cardiol* 2021; **18**: 136–145, doi:10.1038/s41569-020-00463-7.

8. Correll, C. U. *et al.* Prevalence, incidence and mortality from cardiovascular disease in patients with pooled and specific severe mental illness: a large-scale meta-analysis of 3,211,768 patients and 113,383,368 controls. *World Psychiatry* 2017; **16**: 163–180, doi:10.1002/wps.20420.

9. Gaughran, F. *et al.* Randomised control trial of the effectiveness of an integrated psychosocial health promotion intervention aimed at improving health and reducing substance use in established psychosis (IMPaCT). *BMC Psychiatry* 2017; **17**: 413, doi:10.1186/s12888-017-1571-0.

10. Taipale, H. *et al.* 20-year follow-up study of physical morbidity and mortality in relationship to antipsychotic treatment in a nationwide cohort of 62,250 patients with schizophrenia (FIN20). *World Psychiatry* 2020; **19**: 61–68, doi:10.1002/wps.20699.

11. Veeneman, R. R. *et al.* Exploring the relationship between schizophrenia and cardiovascular disease: a genetic correlation and multivariable mendelian randomization study. *Schizophr Bull* 2021; **48**: 463–473, doi:10.1093/schbul/sbab132.

12. Taylor, D. M. *et al. The Maudsley® Prescribing Guidelines in Psychiatry*. 14 edn. (Wiley Blackwell, 2021).

13. National Institute for, H. & Care, E. *Depression in Adults with a Chronic Physical Health Problem* (British Psychological Society, 2010).

14. Cipriani, A. *et al.* Comparative efficacy and acceptability of 21 antidepressant drugs for the acute treatment of adults with major depressive disorder: a systematic review and network meta-analysis. *Lancet* 2018; **391**: 1357–1366, doi:10.1016/S0140-6736(17)32802-7.

15. Hasnain, M. *et al.* Escitalopram and QTc prolongation. *J Psych Neuro* 2013; **38**(4): E11. doi:10.1503/jpn.130055.

16. Rochester, M. P. *et al.* Evaluating the risk of QTc prolongation associated with antidepressant use in older adults: a review of the evidence. *Ther Adv Drug Saf* 2018; **9**: 297–308.

17. Oliva, V. *et al.* Gastrointestinal side effects associated with antidepressant treatments in patients with major depressive disorder: a systematic review and meta-analysis. *Prog Neuro-Psychopharmacol Biol Psychiatry* 2021; **109**: 110266.

18. Cheng, D. *et al.* AHA scientific statement on behalf of the American Heart Association Clinical Pharmacology and Heart Failure and Transplantation Committees of the Council on Clinical Cardiology; Council on Cardiovascular Surgery and Anesthesia; Council on Cardiovascular and Stroke Nursing; and Council on Quality of Care and Outcomes Research Drugs that may cause or exacerbate heart failure: a scientific statement from the American Heart Association. *Circulation* 2016; **134**: 32–69, doi:10.1161/CIR.0000000000000426.

19. Davies, S. J. C. *et al.* Treatment of anxiety and depressive disorders in patients with cardiovascular disease. *Br Med J* 2004; **328**(7445): 939–943.

20. de la Cruz, A. *et al.* Current updates regarding antidepressant prescribing in cardiovascular dysfunction. *Am Coll Cardiology* January 7, 2019. https://www.acc.org/latest-in-cardiology/articles/2019/01/04/07/59/current-updates-regarding-antidepressant-prescribing-in-cv-dysfunction.

21. Mannheimer, B. *et al.* Time-dependent association between selective serotonin reuptake inhibitors and hospitalization due to hyponatremia. *J Psychopharmacol* 2021, doi:10.1177/02698811211001082.

22. Coulter, D. M. *et al.* Antipsychotic drugs and heart muscle disorder in international pharmacovigilance: data mining study. *Br Med J* 2001; **322**: 1207–1209, doi:10.1136/bmj.322.7296.1207.

23. Wu, C. S. *et al.* Antipsychotic drugs and the risk of ventricular arrhythmia and/or sudden cardiac death: a nationwide case 2010; crossover study. *J Am Heart Assoc* 2015; **4**: e001568, doi:10.1161/JAHA.114.001568.

24. Pillinger, T. *et al.* Comparative effects of 18 antipsychotics on metabolic function in patients with schizophrenia, predictors of metabolic dysregulation, and association with psychopathology: a systematic review and network meta-analysis. *Lancet Psychiatry* 2020; **7**: 64–77, doi:10.1016/s2215-0366(19)30416-x.

25. Suter, T. M. *et al.* Trastuzumab-associated cardiac adverse effects in the herceptin adjuvant trial. *J Clin Oncol* 2007; **25**: 3859–3865, doi:10.1200/jco.2006.09.1611.

26. Sweeney, M. *et al.* Understanding and managing cardiac side-effects of second-generation antipsychotics in the treatment of schizophrenia. *BJPsych Advances* 2020; **26**: 26–40, doi:10.1192/bja.2019.49.

27. Whiskey, E. *et al.* Resolution without discontinuation: heart failure during clozapine treatment. *Ther Adv Psychopharmacol* 2020; **10**: doi:10.1177/2045125320924786.

28. Knoph, K. N. *et al.* Clozapine-induced cardiomyopathy and myocarditis monitoring: A systematic review. *Schizophrenia Res* 2018; **199**: 17–30, doi: https://doi.org/10.1016/j.schres.2018.03.006.

29. Page, R. L.'*et al.* Drugs that may cause or exacerbate heart failure. *Circulation* 2016; **134**: e32–e69, doi:doi:10.1161/CIR.0000000000000426.

30. Shah, R. R. Cardiac effects of antiepileptic drugs. *Atlas of Epilepsies* (ed. C. P. Panayiotopoulos) 1479–1486 (Springer London, 2010).

31. Liang, D. *et al.* The relationship between valproate and lamotrigine/levetiracetam use and prognosis in patients with epilepsy and heart failure: a Danish register-based study. *J Card Failure* 2022; **28**: 630–638, doi:10.1016/j.cardfail.2021.07.020.

32. French, J. A. *et al.* FDA safety warning on the cardiac effects of lamotrigine: an advisory from the ad hoc ILAE/AES task force. *Epilepsy Curr* 2021; **21**: 1535759721996344, doi:10.1177/1535759721996344.

33. Owczuk, R. *et al.* Influence of promethazine on cardiac repolarisation: a double-blind, midazolam-controlled study. *Anaesthesia* 2009; **64**: 609–614, doi:10.1111/j.1365-2044.2009.05890.x.

34. Shah, A. *et al.* Diphenhydramine and QT prolongation - A rare cardiac side effect of a drug used in common practice. *J Cardiol Cases* 2015; **12**: 126–129, doi:10.1016/j.jccase.2015.06.002.

35. Husain, Z. *et al.* Diphenhydramine induced QT prolongation and torsade de pointes: An uncommon effect of a common drug. *Cardiology Journal* 2010; **17**: 509–511.

36. Sato, Y. *et al.* Associations of benzodiazepine with adverse prognosis in heart failure patients with insomnia. *J Am Heart Assoc* 2020; **9**: e013982, doi:10.1161/jaha.119.013982.

37. Chuang, C. *et al.* Benzodiazepines in patients with heart failure and reduced ejection fraction. *Acta Cardiologica Sinica* 2022; **38**: 573–583, doi:10.6515/acs.202209_38(5).20220406a.

38. Diez-Quevedo, C. *et al.* Benzodiazepine use and long-term mortality in real-life chronic heart failure outpatients: a cohort analysis. *Psychother Psychosom* 2018; **87**: 372–374, doi:10.1159/000491879.

39. Salamanca-Bautista, P. *et al.* Safety of benzodiazepines in patients with acute heart failure: A propensity score-matching study. *Int J Cardiol* 2023; **382**: 40–45, doi:10.1016/j.ijcard.2023.04.014.

40. Wu, C. K. *et al.* Anti-anxiety drugs use and cardiovascular outcomes in patients with myocardial infarction: a national wide assessment. *Atherosclerosis* 2014; **235**: 496–502, doi:10.1016/j.atherosclerosis.2014.05.918).

41. Howes, L. G. Cardiovascular effects of drugs used to treat Alzheimer's disease. *Drug Saf* 2014; **37**: 391–395, doi:10.1007/s40264-014-0161-z.

42. Hsieh, M. J. *et al.* Association between cholinesterase inhibitors and new-onset heart failure in patients with alzheimer's disease: a nationwide propensity score matching study. *Front Cardiovasc Med* 2022; **9**: 831730, doi:10.3389/fcvm.2022.831730.

43. Rampa, L. *et al.* Potential cardiologic protective effects of acetylcholinesterase inhibitors in patients with mild to moderate dementia. *Am J Cardiol* 2023; **200**: 162–170, doi:10.1016/j.amjcard.2023.05.041.

44. Huang, A. *et al.* Memantine is associated with decreased hospital admissions for heart failure exacerbation, but not arrhythmia: a single-centre study. *J Am Coll Cardiology* 2020; **75**: 1090–1090, doi:doi:10.1016/S0735-1097(20)31717-4.

45. Vaccarino, V. *et al.* Depression and coronary heart disease: 2018 position paper of the ESC working group on coronary pathophysiology and microcirculation. *Eur Heart J* 2019; **41**: 1687–1696, doi:10.1093/eurheartj/ehy913.

46. Carney, R. M. & Freedland, K. E. Depression and coronary heart disease. *Nat Rev Cardiol* 2017; **14**: 145–155, doi:10.1038/nrcardio.2016.181.

47. Nemeroff, C. B. *et al.* Heartache and heartbreak – the link between depression and cardiovascular disease. *Nat Rev Cardiol* 2012; **9**: 526–539, doi:10.1038/nrcardio.2012.91.

48. Berkman, L. F. *et al.* Effects of treating depression and low perceived social support on clinical events after myocardial infarction: the enhancing recovery in coronary heart disease patients (enrichd) randomized trial. *JAMA* 2003; **289**: doi:10.1001/jama.289.23.3106.

49. Glassman, A. H. *et al.* Psychiatric characteristics associated with long-term mortality among 361 patients having an acute coronary syndrome and major depression: seven-year follow-up of SADHART participants. *Arch Gen Psych* 2009; **66**: 1022–1029, doi:10.1001/archgenpsychiatry.2009.121.

50. Jiang, W. *et al.* Characteristics of depression remission and its relation with cardiovascular outcome among patients with chronic heart failure (from the SADHART-CHF Study). *Am J Cardiol* 2011; **107**: 545–551, doi:10.1016/j.amjcard.2010.10.013.

51. de Jonge, P. *et al.* Nonresponse to treatment for depression following myocardial infarction: association with subsequent cardiac events. *Am J Psychiatry* 2007; **164**: 1371–1378, doi:10.1176/appi.ajp.2007.06091492.

52. Grace, S. L. *et al.* Prospective examination of anxiety persistence and its relationship to cardiac symptoms and recurrent cardiac events. *Psychother Psychosom* 2004; **73**: 344–352, doi:10.1159/000080387.

53. Roest, A. M. *et al.* Anxiety and risk of incident coronary heart disease. *J Am Coll Cardiology* 2010; **56**: 38–46, doi:doi:10.1016/j.jacc.2010.03.034.

54. Roest, A. M. *et al.* Prognostic association of anxiety post myocardial infarction with mortality and new cardiac events: a meta-analysis. *Psychosom Med* 2010; **72**: 563–569, doi:10.1097/PSY.0b013e3181dbff97.

55. Watkins, L. L. *et al.* Association of anxiety and depression with all-cause mortality in individuals with coronary heart disease. *J Am Heart Assoc* 2013; **2**: e000068, doi:10.1161/jaha.112.000068.

56. Farquhar, J. M. *et al.* Treatment of anxiety in patients with coronary heart disease: a systematic review. *Psychosomatics* 2018; **59**: 318–332, doi:https://doi.org/10.1016/j.psym.2018.03.008.

57. Rossom, R. C. *et al.* Cardiovascular risk for patients with and without schizophrenia, schizoaffective disorder, or bipolar disorder. *J Am Heart Assoc* 2022; **11**: e021444, doi:10.1161/jaha.121.021444.

58. To, B. T. *et al.* Coronary artery disease in patients with severe mental illness. *Interven Cardiology* 2023; **18**: e16, doi:10.15420/icr.2022.31.

59. J.C, N. *et al.* Treatment of major depression with nortriptyline and paroxetine in patients with ischemic heart disease. *Am J Psychiatry* 1999; 156.

60. Roose, S. P. *et al.* Comparison of paroxetine and nortriptyline in depressed patients with ischemic heart disease. *JAMA* 1998; 279, doi:10.1001/jama.279.4.287.

61. Van Melle, J. P. *et al.* Effects of antidepressant treatment following myocardial infarction. *Br J Psych* 2007; **190**: doi:10.1192/bjp.bp.106.028647.

62. Parissis, J. T. *et al.* Combined prognostic value of self-rating depression scores and plasma b-type natriuretic peptide in hospitalized patients with chronic heart failure. *International Journal of Cardiology* 2007; **116**: no. suppe. 16.

63. Yuet, W. C. *et al.* Selective serotonin reuptake inhibitor use and risk of gastrointestinal and intracranial bleeding. *J Osteo Med* 2019; **119**: 10–111, doi:doi:10.7556/jaoa.2019.016.

64. Yu, Z. H. *et al.* Use of antipsychotics and risk of myocardial infarction: a systematic review and meta-analysis. *Br J Clin Psych* 2016; **82**: 624–632, doi:10.1111/bcp.12985.

65. Papola, D. *et al.* Antipsychotic use and risk of life-threatening medical events: umbrella review of observational studies. *Acta Cardiologica Scandinavica* 2019; **140**, 227–243, doi:10.1111/acps.13066.

66. Rotella, F. *et al.* Long-term metabolic and cardiovascular effects of antipsychotic drugs. A meta-analysis of randomized controlled trials. *Eur Neuropsychopharmacol* 2020; **32**: 56–65, doi:https://doi.org/10.1016/j.euroneuro.2019.12.118.

67. Zivkovic, S. *et al.* Antipsychotic drug use and risk of stroke and myocardial infarction: a systematic review and meta-analysis. *BMC Psychiatry* 2019; **19**: 189, doi:10.1186/s12888-019-2177-5.

68. Shaper, A. G. *et al.* Risk factors for ischaemic heart disease: the prospective phase of the British Regional Heart Study. *J Epid Comm Health* 1985; **39**: 197–209, doi:10.1136/jech.39.3.197.

69. Lin, S.-T. *et al.* Association between antipsychotic use and risk of acute myocardial infarction. *Circulation* 2014; **130**: 235–243, doi:10.1161/CIRCULATIONAHA.114.008779.

70. Tsai, S.-Y. *et al.* The association between carotid atherosclerosis and treatment with lithium and antipsychotics in patients with bipolar disorder. *Aus & NZ J Psychiatry* 2020; **54**: 1125–1134, doi:10.1177/0004867420952551.

71. Ahrens, B. *et al.* Excess cardiovascular and suicide mortality of affective disorders may be reduced by lithium prophylaxis. *J Aff Disord* 1995; **33**: 67–75, doi:10.1016/0165-0327(94)00074-j.

72. Mehta, N. *et al.* Lithium-induced electrocardiographic changes: a complete review. *Clin Cardiology* 2017; **40**: 1363–1367, doi: https://doi.org/10.1002/clc.22822.

CHAPTER 1

73. LoPinto-Khoury, C. *et al.* Antiepileptic drugs and markers of vascular risk. *Current Treat Opt Neurology* 2010; **12**: 300–308, doi:10.1007/s11940-010-0080-y.

74. Mintzer, S. *et al.* Hyperlipidemia in patients newly treated with anticonvulsants: A population study. *Epilepsia* 2020; **61**: 259–266, doi:10.1111/epi.16420.

75. Renoux, C. *et al.* Antiepileptic drugs and the risk of ischaemic stroke and myocardial infarction: a population-based cohort study. *BMJ Open* 2015; **5**: e008365, doi:10.1136/bmjopen-2015-008365.

76. Olesen, J. B. *et al.* Valproate attenuates the risk of myocardial infarction in patients with epilepsy: a nationwide cohort study. *Pharmacoepidemiol Drug Saf* 2011; **20**: 146–153, doi:10.1002/pds.2073.

77. Olesen, J. B. *et al.* Effects of epilepsy and selected antiepileptic drugs on risk of myocardial infarction, stroke, and death in patients with or without previous stroke: a nationwide cohort study. *Pharmacoepidemiol Drug Saf* 2011; **20**: 964–971, doi: https://doi.org/10.1002/pds.2186.

78. Parsons, K. *et al.* Glycemic and serum lipid control in patients with painful diabetic peripheral neuropathy treated with pregabalin. *J Diabetes Complications* 2017; **31**: 489–493, doi:10.1016/j.jdiacomp.2016.03.019.

79. Lee-Lane, E. *et al.* Epilepsy, antiepileptic drugs, and the risk of major cardiovascular events. *Epilepsia* 2021; **62**: 1604–1616, doi: https://doi.org/10.1111/epi.16930.

80. Liu, S. *et al.* Use of benzodiazepine and Z-drugs and mortality in older adults after myocardial infarction. *Int J Geriatr Psychiatry* 2023; **38**: e5861, doi:10.1002/gps.5861.

81. Nordström, P. *et al.* The use of cholinesterase inhibitors and the risk of myocardial infarction and death: a nationwide cohort study in subjects with Alzheimer's disease. *Eur Heart J* 2013; **34**: 2585–2591, doi:10.1093/eurheartj/eht182.

82. Khuanjing, T. *et al.* The effects of acetylcholinesterase inhibitors on the heart in acute myocardial infarction and heart failure: From cells to patient reports. *Acta Physiologica (Oxf)* 2020; **228**: e13396, doi:10.1111/apha.13396.

83. Jannesar, K. *et al.* Cardioprotective effects of memantine in myocardial ischemia: Ex vivo and in vivo studies. *Eur J Pharmacology* 2020; **882**: 173277, doi:10.1016/j.ejphar.2020.173277.

84. Huang, W.-C. *et al.* Association between recently raised anticholinergic burden and risk of acute cardiovascular events: nationwide case-case-time-control study. *BMJ* 2023; **382**: e076045, doi:10.1136/bmj-2023-076045.

85. Craig, M. Blood-pressure in the insane. *Lancet* 1898; **151**: 1742–1747, doi: https://doi.org/10.1016/S0140-6736(01)78434-6.

86. Meng, L. *et al.* Depression increases the risk of hypertension incidence: a meta-analysis of prospective cohort studies. *J Hypertension* 2012; **30**: 842–851, doi:10.1097/HJH.0b013e32835080b7.

87. Taylor, W. D. *et al.* The vascular depression hypothesis: mechanisms linking vascular disease with depression. *Mol Psychiatry* 2013; **18**: 963–974, doi:10.1038/mp.2013.20.

88. Hassoun, L. *et al.* Association between chronic stress and blood pressure: findings from the German Health Interview and Examination Survey for Adults 2008–2011. *Psychosom Med* 2015; **77**: 575–582, doi:10.1097/psy.0000000000000183.

89. Schaare, H. L. *et al.* Associations between mental health, blood pressure and the development of hypertension. *Nature Communications* 2023; **14**: 1953, doi:10.1038/s41467-023-37579-6.

90. Markovitz, J. H. *et al.* Psychological predictors of hypertension in the Framingham Study: is there tension in hypertension? *JAMA* 1993; **270**: 2439–2443, doi:10.1001/jama.1993.03510200045030.

91. Jonas, B. S. *et al.* Are symptoms of anxiety and depression risk factors for hypertension? Longitudinal evidence from the National Health and Nutrition Examination Survey I Epidemiologic Follow-up Study. *Arch Fam Med* 1997; **6**: 43–49, doi:10.1001/archfami.6.1.43.

92. Pan, Y. *et al.* Association between anxiety and hypertension: a systematic review and meta-analysis of epidemiological studies. *Neuropsychiatr Dis Treat* 2015; **11**: 1121–1130, doi:10.2147/ndt.S77710.

93. Hamer, M. *et al.* Hypertension awareness and psychological distress. *Hypertension* 2010; **56**: 547–550, doi:10.1161/hypertensionaha.110.153775.).

94. Yasunari, K. *et al.* Anxiety-induced plasma norepinephrine augmentation increases reactive oxygen species formation by monocytes in essential hypertension. *Am J Hypertens* 2006; **19**: 573–578, doi:10.1016/j.amjhyper.2005.10.027.

95. Mitchell, A. J. *et al.* Prevalence of metabolic syndrome and metabolic abnormalities in schizophrenia and related disorders – a systematic review and meta-analysis. *Schizophr Bull* 2013; **39**: 306–318, doi:10.1093/schbul/sbr148.

96. Gardner-Sood, P. *et al.* Cardiovascular risk factors and metabolic syndrome in people with established psychotic illnesses: baseline data from the IMPaCT randomized controlled trial. *Psychol Med* 2015; **45**: 2619–2629, doi:10.1017/s0033291715000562.

97. Goldstein, B. I. *et al.* Cardiovascular disease and hypertension among adults with bipolar I disorder in the United States. *Bipolar Disord* 2009; **11**: 657–662, doi:10.1111/j.1399-5618.2009.00735.x.

98. Ayerbe, L. *et al.* Hypertension risk and clinical care in patients with bipolar disorder or schizophrenia; a systematic review and meta-analysis. *J Aff Disord* 2018; **225**: 665–670, doi:10.1016/j.jad.2017.09.002.

99. Tsao, W. Y. *et al.* Risk of cardiometabolic diseases among siblings of patients with bipolar disorder. *J Aff Disord* 2019; **253**: 171–175, doi:10.1016/j.jad.2019.04.094.).

100. Sudarshan, Y. *et al.* Hypertension and psychosis. *Postgraduate Medical Journal* 2022; **99**: 411–415, doi:10.1136/postgradmedj-2021-141386.

101. Dawood, T. *et al.* Response to depression and blodd pressure control: all antidepressants are not the same. *Hypertension* 2009; **54**.

102. Licht, C. M. M. *et al.* Depression is associated with decreased blood pressure, but antidepressant use increases the risk for hypertension. *Hypertension* 2009; **53**: doi:10.1161/HYPERTENSIONAHA.108.126698.

103. Feighner, J. P. Cardiovascular safety in depressed patients: Focus on venlafaxine. *J Clin Psychiatry* 1995; **56**.

104. Zhong, Z. *et al.* A meta-analysis of effects of selective serotonin reuptake inhibitors on blood pressure in depression treatment: Outcomes from placebo and serotonin and noradrenaline reuptake inhibitor controlled trials. *Neuropsych Dis Treatment* 2017; **13**: doi:10.2147/NDT.S141832.

105. Jette, N., Veregin, T. & Guberman, A. Carbamazepine-induced hypertension. *Neurology* 2002; **59**: 275–276, doi:10.1212/wnl.59.2.275.

106. Sivananthan, M. *et al.* Valproate induced hypertensive urgency. *Case Rep Psychiatry* 2016; 1458548, doi:10.1155/2016/1458548.

107. Micromedex®. in *Micromedex®* V. 2.0 (2020).

108. McGowan, N. M. *et al.* Blood pressure in bipolar disorder: evidence of elevated pulse pressure and associations between mean pressure and mood instability. *Inter J Bipolar Disord* 2021; **9**: 5, doi:10.1186/s40345-020-00209-x.

109. Howarth, S. *et al.* Action of promethazine on systemic blood pressure, pulmonary artery pressure and pulmonary bloodflow. *Br Med J* 1954; **2**: 1266–1267, doi:10.1136/bmj.2.4899.1266.

110. Mackmull, G. The influence of intravenously administered benadryl on blood pressure and electrocardiogram. *J Allergy* 1948; **19**: 365–370, doi:10.1016/0021-8707(48)90030-6.

111. Mendelson, N. *et al.* Benzodiazepine consumption is associated with lower blood pressure in ambulatory blood pressure monitoring (ABPM): retrospective analysis of 4938 ABPMs. *Am J Hypertension* 2018; **31**: 431–437, doi:10.1093/ajh/hpx188.

112. Solanki, B. *et al.* Benzodiazepines reduce blood pressure in short term: a systematic review and meta-analysis. *Curr Hypertension Rep* 2023; **25**: 335–341, doi:10.1007/s11906-023-01256-2.

113. van Marum, R. J. Update on the use of memantine in Alzheimer's disease. *Neuropsych Dis Treatment* 2009; **5**: 237–247, doi:10.2147/ndt.s4048.

114. Hackett, M. L. *et al.* Part I: frequency of depression after stroke: an updated systematic review and meta-analysis of observational studies. *Inter J Stroke* 2014; **9**: 1017–1025.

115. Towfighi, A. *et al.* Poststroke depression: a scientific statement for healthcare professionals from the American Heart Association/American Stroke Association. *Stroke* 2017; **48**: e30–e43, doi:10.1161/str.0000000000000113.

116. Ayerbe, L. *et al.* The natural history of depression up to 15 years after stroke. *Stroke* 2013; **44**: 1105–1110, doi:doi:10.1161/STROKEAHA.111.679340.).

117. Knapp, P. *et al.* Frequency of anxiety after stroke: An updated systematic review and meta-analysis of observational studies. *Int J Stroke* 2020; **15**: 244–255, doi:10.1177/1747493019896958.).

118. Wright, F. *et al.* Factors associated with poststroke anxiety: a systematic review and meta-analysis. *Stroke Res Treatment* 2017: 2124743, doi:10.1155/2017/2124743.

119. Knapp, P. *et al.* Interventions for treating anxiety after stroke. *Cochrane Database Syst Rev* 2017; **5**, Cd008860, doi:10.1002/14651858.CD008860.pub3.).

120. Li, W. *et al.* Anxiety in patients with acute ischemic stroke: risk factors and effects on functional status. *Front Psychiatry* 2019; **10**: 257, doi:10.3389/fpsyt.2019.00257.

121. Li, M. *et al.* Schizophrenia and risk of stroke: A meta-analysis of cohort studies. *Inter J Cardiology* 2014; **173**: 588–590, doi:https://doi.org/10.1016/j.ijcard.2014.03.101.

122. Fleetwood, K. *et al.* Association of severe mental illness with stroke outcomes and process-of-care quality indicators: nationwide cohort study. *Br J Psych* 2022; **221**: 394–401, doi:10.1192/bjp.2021.120.

123. Prieto, M. L. *et al.* Risk of myocardial infarction and stroke in bipolar disorder: a systematic review and exploratory meta-analysis. *Acta Psychiatr Scand* 2014; **130**: 342–353, doi:10.1111/acps.12293.

124. Yung, N. C. L. *et al.* Mortality in patients with schizophrenia admitted for incident ischemic stroke: A population-based cohort study. *Eur Neuropsychopharmacol* 2020; **31**: 152–157, doi: https://doi.org/10.1016/j.euroneuro.2019.12.107.

125. Matheson, E. *et al.* Abstract WMP54: Stroke secondary prevention care in persons with schizophrenia. *Stroke* 2022; **53**: doi:10.1161/str.53.suppl_1.WMP54.

126. Kapral, M. K. *et al.* Stroke care and case fatality in people with and without schizophrenia: a retrospective cohort study. *BMJ Open* 2021; **11**: e044766, doi:10.1136/bmjopen-2020-044766.

127. Bongiorno, D. M. *et al.* Comorbid psychiatric disease is associated with lower rates of thrombolysis in ischemic stroke. *Stroke* 2018; **49**: 738–740, doi:10.1161/strokeaha.117.020295.

128. Willers, C. *et al.* The association of pre-stroke psychosis and post-stroke levels of health, resource utilization, and care process: a register-based study. *Front Neurol* 2018; **9**: 1042, doi:10.3389/fneur.2018.01042.

129. Bongiorno, D. M. *et al.* Patients with stroke and psychiatric comorbidities have lower carotid revascularization rates. *Neurology* 2019; **92**: e2514–e2521, doi:10.1212/wnl.0000000000007565.

130. Mead, G. E. *et al.* Selective serotonin reuptake inhibitors for stroke recovery. *JAMA* 2013; **310**: 1066–1067, doi:10.1001/jama.2013.107828.).

131. Jorge, R. E. *et al.* Mortality and poststroke depression: a placebo-controlled trial of antidepressants. *Am J Psychiatry* 2003; **160**: 1823–1829, doi:10.1176/appi.ajp.160.10.1823.

132. Krivoy, A. *et al.* Low adherence to antidepressants is associated with increased mortality following stroke: A large nationally representative cohort study. *Eur Neuropsychopharmacol* 2017; **27**: doi:10.1016/j.euroneuro.2017.08.428.

133. Li, X. *et al.* Comparative efficacy of nine antidepressants in treating Chinese patients with post-stroke depression: a network meta-analysis. *J Aff Disord* 2020; **266**.

134. Niedermaier, N. *et al.* Prevention and treatment of poststroke depression with mirtazapine in patients with acute stroke. *J Clin Psych* 2004; **65**, doi:10.4088/JCP.v65n1206.

135. Chen, W. Y. *et al.* Antipsychotic medications and stroke in schizophrenia: A case-crossover study. *PLoS One* 2017; **12**: e0179424, doi:10.1371/journal.pone.0179424.

136. Hsu, W. T. *et al.* Antipsychotics and the risk of cerebrovascular accident: a systematic review and meta-analysis of observational studies. *J Am Med Dir Assoc* 2017; **18**: 692–699, doi:10.1016/j.jamda.2017.02.020.

137. Chen, B. *et al.* The neuroprotective mechanism of lithium after ischaemic stroke. *Communications Biology* 2022; **5**: 105, doi:10.1038/s42003-022-03051-2.).

138. Sun, Y. R. *et al*. Lithium carbonate in a poststroke population: exploratory analyses of neuroanatomical and cognitive outcomes. *J Clin Psychopharmacol* 2019; **39**: 67–71, doi:10.1097/jcp.0000000000000981.

139. Almeida, O. P. *et al*. Lithium and stroke recovery: a systematic review and meta-analysis of stroke models in rodents and human data. *Stroke* 2022; **53**: 2935–2944, doi:10.1161/strokeaha.122.039203.

140. Chen, P. H. *et al*. Mood stabilisers and risk of stroke in bipolar disorder. *Br J Psych* 2019; **215**: 409–414, doi:10.1192/bjp.2018.203.

141. Lan, C. C. *et al*. A reduced risk of stroke with lithium exposure in bipolar disorder: a population-based retrospective cohort study. *Bipolar Disorders* 2015; **17**: 705–714, doi:10.1111/bdi.12336.

142. Brookes, R. L. *et al*. Sodium valproate, a histone deacetylase inhibitor, is associated with reduced stroke risk after previous ischemic stroke or transient ischemic attack. *Stroke* 2018; **49**: 54–61, doi:10.1161/strokeaha.117.016674.

143. Larsson, D. *et al*. Association between antiseizure drug monotherapy and mortality for patients with poststroke epilepsy. *JAMA Neurology* 2022; **79**: 169–175, doi:10.1001/jamaneurol.2021.4584.

144. Karlsson Lind, L. *et al*. Antiepileptic medicines in men and women with stroke in Sweden, a registry-based study. *Health Science Reports* 2021; **4**: e405, doi: https://doi.org/10.1002/hsr2.405.

145. Kugler, C. *et al*. Pregabalin improves axon regeneration and motor outcome in a rodent stroke model. *Brain Communications* 2022; **4**: doi:10.1093/braincomms/fcac170.

146. Guo, S. *et al*. Chlorpromazine and promethazine (C+P) reduce brain injury after ischemic stroke through the PKC-δ/NOX/MnSOD pathway. *Mediators Inflamm* 2022: 6886752, doi:10.1155/2022/6886752.

147. Liu, J. *et al*. Gamma aminobutyric acid (GABA) receptor agonists for acute stroke. *Cochrane Database Syst Rev* 2018; **10**: Cd009622, doi:10.1002/14651858.CD009622.pub5.

148. Colin, O. *et al*. Preadmission use of benzodiazepines and stroke outcomes: the biostroke prospective cohort study. *BMJ Open* 2019; **9**: e022720, doi:10.1136/bmjopen-2018-022720.

149. Huang, W. S. *et al*. Benzodiazepine use and risk of stroke: a retrospective population-based cohort study. *Psychiatry Clin Neurosci* 2014; **68**: 255–262, doi:10.1111/pcn.12117.

150. Lin, S.-M. *et al*. Association between benzodiazepine use and risks of chronic-onset poststroke pneumonia: a population-based cohort study. *BMJ Open* 2019; **9**: e024180, doi:10.1136/bmjopen-2018-024180.).

151. Moura, L. M. V. R. *et al*. No short-term mortality from benzodiazepine use post-acute ischemic stroke after accounting for bias. *J Clin Epid* 2023; **154**: 136–145, doi: https://doi.org/10.1016/j.jclinepi.2022.12.013.).

152. Lin, Y. T. *et al*. Association between acetylcholinesterase inhibitors and risk of stroke in patients with dementia. *Sci Rep* 2016; **6**: 29266, doi:10.1038/srep29266.).

153. Kim, J. O. *et al*. Effect of acetylcholinesterase inhibitors on post-stroke cognitive impairment and vascular dementia: A meta-analysis. *PLoS One* 2020; **15**: e0227820, doi:10.1371/journal.pone.0227820.).

154. Barfejani, A. H. *et al*. Donepezil in the treatment of ischemic stroke: Review and future perspective. *Life Sci* 2020; **263**: 118575, doi:10.1016/j.lfs.2020.118575.

155. Pichardo-Rojas, D. *et al*. Memantine as a neuroprotective agent in ischemic stroke: Preclinical and clinical analysis. *Front Neurosci* 2023; **17**: 1096372, doi:10.3389/fnins.2023.1096372.).

156. Al-Hamed, F. S. *et al*. Acetylcholinesterase inhibitors and risk of bleeding and acute ischemic events in non-hypertensive Alzheimer's patients. *Alzheimers Dement (N Y)* 2021; **7**, e12184, doi:10.1002/trc2.12184.

157. Kim, Y. G. *et al*. Association of depression with atrial fibrillation in South Korean adults. *JAMA Network Open* 2022; **5**: e2141772–e2141772, doi:10.1001/jamanetworkopen.2021.41772.

158. Bae, N. Y. *et al*. Impact of mental disorders on the risk of atrial fibrillation in patients with diabetes mellitus: a nationwide population-based study. *Cardiovasc Diabetol* 2022; **21**: 251, doi:10.1186/s12933-022-01682-7.

159. Ai, Y. *et al*. Atrial fibrillation and depression: A bibliometric analysis from 2001 to 2021. *Front Cardiovas Med* 2022; **9**, doi:10.3389/fcvm.2022.775329.

160. Zhuo, C. *et al*. Depression and recurrence of atrial fibrillation after catheter ablation: a meta-analysis of cohort studies. *J Aff Disord* 2020; **271**: 27–32, doi:10.1016/j.jad.2020.03.118.

161. Frasure-Smith, N. *et al*. Elevated depression symptoms predict long-term cardiovascular mortality in patients with atrial fibrillation and heart failure. *Circulation* 2009; **120**: 134–140, 133p following 140, doi:10.1161/circulationaha.109.851675.

162. Lombardi, N. *et al*. Adherence to triple-free-drug combination therapies among patients with cardiovascular disease. *Am J Cardiology* 2020; **125**: 1429–1435, doi:10.1016/j.amjcard.2020.01.036.

163. Teppo, K. *et al*. Mental health conditions and risk of first-ever ischaemic stroke and death in patients with incident atrial fibrillation: A nationwide cohort study. *Eur J Clin Investigation* 2022; **52**: e13801, doi:10.1111/eci.13801.

164. Severino, P. *et al*. Triggers for atrial fibrillation: the role of anxiety. *Cardiol Res Practice* 2019: 1208505, doi:10.1155/2019/1208505.).

165. Eaker, E. D. *et al*. Tension and anxiety and the prediction of the 10-year incidence of coronary heart disease, atrial fibrillation, and total mortality: the framingham offspring study. *Psychosom Med* 2005; **67**: 692–696, doi:10.1097/01.psy.0000174050.87193.96.

166. Ahn, H. J. *et al*. Increased risk of incident atrial fibrillation in young adults with mental disorders: A nationwide population-based study. *Heart Rhythm* 2023; **20**: 365–373, doi:10.1016/j.hrthm.2022.12.019.

167. Treur, J. L. *et al*. Associations of schizophrenia with arrhythmic disorders and electrocardiogram traits: an in-depth genetic exploration of population samples. *medRxiv*, 2023, doi:10.1101/2023.05.21.23290286.

168. Teppo, K. *et al*. Mental health conditions and use of rhythm control therapies in patients with atrial fibrillation: a nationwide cohort study. *BMJ Open* 2022; **12**: e059759, doi:10.1136/bmjopen-2021-059759.

169. Højen, A. A. *et al.* Disparities in oral anticoagulation initiation in patients with schizophrenia and atrial fibrillation: A nationwide cohort study. *Br J Clin Pharmacol* 2022; **88**: 3847–3855, doi:10.1111/bcp.15337.

170. Fenger-Grøn, M. *et al.* Association between bipolar disorder or schizophrenia and oral anticoagulation use in danish adults with incident or prevalent atrial fibrillation. *JAMA Netw Open* 2021; **4**: e2110096, doi:10.1001/jamanetworkopen.2021.10096.

171. Teppo, K. *et al.* Mental health conditions and nonpersistence of direct oral anticoagulant use in patients with incident atrial fibrillation: a nationwide cohort study. *J Am Heart Assoc* 2022; **11**: e024119, doi:10.1161/jaha.121.024119.

172. Søgaard, M. *et al.* Atrial fibrillation in patients with severe mental disorders and the risk of stroke, fatal thromboembolic events and bleeding: a nationwide cohort study. *BMJ Open* 2017; **7**: e018209, doi:10.1136/bmjopen-2017-018209.

173. Lapi, F. *et al.* The use of antidepressants and the risk of chronic atrial fibrillation. *J Clin Pharmacol* 2015; **55**: 423–430, doi:10.1002/jcph.435.

174. Yusuf, S. *et al.* 5-hydroxytryptamine and atrial fibrillation: how significant is this piece in the puzzle? *J Cardiovasc Electrophysiol* 2003; **14**: 209–214.

175. Fu, Y. *et al.* Association of depression, antidepressants with atrial fibrillation risk: a systemic review and meta-analysis. *Front Cardiovasc Med* 2022; **9**: 897622, doi:10.3389/fcvm.2022.897622.

176. Fenger-Grøn, M. *et al.* Depression, antidepressants, and the risk of non-valvular atrial fibrillation: A nationwide Danish matched cohort study. *Eur J Prev Cardiol* 2019; **26**: 187–195, doi:10.1177/2047487318811184.

177. Garg, P. K. *et al.* Negative affect and risk of atrial fibrillation: MESA. *J Am Heart Assoc* 2019; **8**: e010603, doi:10.1161/jaha.118.010603.

178. Cao, Y. *et al.* Associations of antidepressants with atrial fibrillation and ventricular arrhythmias: a systematic review and meta-analysis. *Front Cardiovasc Med* 2022; **9**: 840452, doi:10.3389/fcvm.2022.840452.

179. Pacher, P. *et al.* Speculations on difference between tricyclic and selective serotonin reuptake inhibitor antidepressants on their cardiac effects. Is there any? *Curr Med Chem* 1999; **6**: 469–480.

180. D'Urso, G. *et al.* Aripiprazole-induced atrial fibrillation in a patient with concomitant risk factors. *Exp Clin Psychopharmacol* 2018; **26**: 509–513, doi:10.1037/pha0000219.

181. Stefatos, A. *et al.* Atrial fibrillation and injected aripiprazole: a case report. *Innov Clin Neurosci* 2018; **15**: 43–45.

182. Çam, B. *et al.* Clozapine and olanzapine associated atrial fibrillation: a case report. *Turk Psikiyatri Derg* 2015; **26**: 221–226.

183. Low, R. A. *et al.* Clozapine induced atrial fibrillation. *J Clin Psychopharmacol* 1998; **18**: 170, doi:10.1097/00004714-199804000-00010.

184. Waters, B. M. *et al.* Olanzapine-associated new-onset atrial fibrillation. *J Clin Psychopharmacol* 2008; **28**: 354–355, doi:10.1097/JCP.0b013e318173082c.

185. Schneider, R. A. *et al.* Apparent seizure and atrial fibrillation associated with paliperidone. *Am J Health Syst Pharm* 2008; **65**: 2122–2125, doi:10.2146/ajhp070615.).

186. Chou, R. H. *et al.* Antipsychotic treatment is associated with risk of atrial fibrillation: A nationwide nested case-control study. *Int J Cardiol* 2017; **227**: 134–140, doi:10.1016/j.ijcard.2016.11.185.

187. Embi, A. A. *et al.* An endocrine hypothesis for the genesis of atrial fibrillation: the hypothalamic-pituitary-adrenal axis response to stress and glycogen accumulation in atrial tissues. *N Am J Med Sci* 2014; **6**: 586–590, doi:10.4103/1947-2714.145478.

188. Polcwiartek, C. *et al.* Electrocardiogram characteristics and their association with psychotropic drugs among patients with schizophrenia. *Schizophr Bull* 2020; **46**: 354–362, doi:10.1093/schbul/sbz064.

189. Davutoglu, V. *et al.* Valproic acid as a cause of transient atrio-ventricular conduction block episodes. *J Atr Fibrillation* 2017; **9**: 1520, doi:10.4022/jafib.1520.

190. Diserens, L. *et al.* Lithium-induced ECG modifications: navigating from acute coronary syndrome to Brugada syndrome. *BMJ Case Reports* 2021; **14**: doi:10.1136/bcr-2021-241555.

191. Chilkoti, G. *et al.* Could pregabalin premedication predispose to perioperative atrial fibrillation in patients with sepsis? *Saudi J Anaesthesia* 2014; **8**: S115–116, doi:10.4103/1658-354x.144096

192. Laville, M. A. *et al.* Should we care about pregabalin for elderly patients with a history of cardiac dysrhythmia? *Revue de Médecine Interne* 2008; **29**: 152–154, doi:10.1016/j.revmed.2007.07.009.

193. Ortiz de Landaluce, L. *et al.* Gabapentin and pregabalin and risk of atrial fibrillation in the elderly: a population-based cohort study in an electronic prescription database. *Drug Saf* 2018; **41**: 1325–1331, doi:10.1007/s40264-018-0695-6.

194. Sessa, M. *et al.* The risk of fractures, acute myocardial infarction, atrial fibrillation and ventricular arrhythmia in geriatric patients exposed to promethazine. *Expert Opin Drug Saf* 2020; **19**: 349–357, doi:10.1080/14740338.2020.1711882.

195. Mandyam, M. C. *et al.* The QT interval and risk of incident atrial fibrillation. *Heart Rhythm* 2013; **10**: 1562–1568, doi:10.1016/j.hrthm.2013.07.023.

196. Bishara, D. *et al.* Anticholinergic effect on cognition (AEC) of drugs commonly used in older people. *Int J Geriatr Psychiatry* 2017; **32**: 650–656, doi:10.1002/gps.4507.

197. Hu, X. *et al.* Hypnotics use is associated with elevated incident atrial fibrillation: a propensity-score matched analysis of cohort study. *J Pers Med* 2022; **12**: doi:10.3390/jpm12101645.

198. Hung, C. Y. *et al.* Falls and atrial fibrillation in elderly patients. *Acta Cardiol Sin* 2013; **29**: 436–443.

199. Jurin, I. *et al.* The risk of falling and consequences of falling in patients with atrial fibrillation receiving different types of anticoagulant. *Drugs Aging* 2021; **38**: 417–425, doi:10.1007/s40266-021-00843-9.

200. Wang, D. *et al.* Electrocardiogram Changes of donepezil administration in elderly patients with ischemic heart disease. *Cardiol Res Pract* 2018: 9141320, doi:10.1155/2018/9141320.

201. Huang, Y. *et al.* Comparative risk of cardiac arrhythmias associated with acetylcholinesterase inhibitors used in treatment of dementias – A narrative review. *Pharmacol Res Perspect* 2020; **8**: e00622, doi:10.1002/prp2.622.

CHAPTER 1

202. Xie, D. *et al.* Memantine targets glutamate receptors in atrial cardiomyocytes to prevent and treat atrial fibrillation. *Cell Discov* 2022; 8: 76, doi:10.1038/s41421-022-00429-8.

203. Labos, C. *et al.* Risk of bleeding associated with combined use of selective serotonin reuptake inhibitors and antiplatelet therapy following acute myocardial infarction. *Cmaj* 2011; 183: 1835–1843, doi:10.1503/cmaj.100912.

204. Machado, C. M. *et al.* Impact of selective serotonin-reuptake inhibitors in hemorrhagic risk in anticoagulated patients taking non-vitamin K antagonist anticoagulants: a systematic review and meta-analysis. *J Clin Psychopharmacol* 2023; 43: 267–272, doi:10.1097/jcp.0000000000001684.

205. Stockley, I. H. *Stockley's Drug Interactions*. Pharmaceutical Press (2008).

206. Spaans, E. *et al.* The effects of mirtazapine on steady state prothrombin time during warfarin therapy. *Pharmacol Toxicol* 2001; 89: 80.

207. Norton, J. *et al.* Mirtazapine-induced warfarin toxicity. *Primary Psychiatry* 2002; 9: 30–31.

208. Nishimura, H. *et al.* A case with the increased PT-INR after the addition of mirtazapine to warfarin therapy. *Seishin Shinkeigaku Zasshi* 2015; 117: 820–825.

209. Chang, K. H. *et al.* Major bleeding risk in patients with non-valvular atrial fibrillation concurrently taking direct oral anticoagulants and antidepressants. *Front Aging Neurosci* 2022; 14: 791285, doi:10.3389/fnagi.2022.791285

210. Verdel, B. M. *et al.* Use of serotonergic drugs and the risk of bleeding. *Clin Pharmacol Therapeutics* 2011; 89: 89–96, doi: https://doi.org/10.1038/clpt.2010.240.

211. Chen, C. M. *et al.* Major bleeding risk in atrial fibrillation patients co-medicated with non-vitamin K oral anticoagulants and antipsychotics. *Front Pharmacol* 2022; 13: 819878, doi:10.3389/fphar.2022.819878.

212. Parker, C. *et al.* Antipsychotic drugs and risk of venous thromboembolism: nested case-control study. *BMJ* 2010; 341: c4245, doi:10.1136/bmj.c4245.

213. Loiseau, P. Sodium valproate, platelet dysfunction, and bleeding. *Epilepsia* 1981; 22: 141–146, doi: https://doi.org/10.1111/j.1528-1157.1981.tb04094.x.

214. Fajardo, A. *et al.* Valproic acid and the risk of perioperative bleeding. Case report and literature review. *Col J Anesthesiol* 2013; 41: 61–64, doi: https://doi.org/10.1016/j.rcae.2012.07.007.

215. Post, D. S. *et al.* Assessment of need for hemostatic evaluation in patients taking valproic acid: A retrospective cross-sectional study. *PLOS ONE* 2022; 17: e0264351, doi:10.1371/journal.pone.0264351.

216. Shan, J. *et al.* Prevalence of heavy menstrual bleeding and its associated cognitive risks and predictive factors in women with severe mental disorders. *Front Pharmacol* 2022; 13: 904908, doi:10.3389/fphar.2022.904908.

217. Sleiman, C. *et al.* Fatal Pulmonary hemorrhage during high-dose valproate monotherapy. *Chest* 2000; 117: 613, doi: https://doi.org/10.1378/chest.117.2.613.

218. Johnston, J. P. *et al.* Valproic acid-induced thrombocytopenia-related spontaneous systemic Bleeding. *Am J Case Rep* 2020; 21: e927830, doi:10.12659/ajcr.927830.

219. Chen, H. F. *et al.* Valproic acid-associated low fibrinogen and delayed intracranial hemorrhage: case report and mini literature review. *Drug Des Devel Ther* 2013; 7: 767–770, doi:10.2147/dddt.S47718.

220. Steffel, J. *et al.* The 2018 European Heart Rhythm Association practical guide on the use of non-vitamin K antagonist oral anticoagulants in patients with atrial fibrillation. *Eur Heart J* 2018; 39: 1330–1393, doi:10.1093/eurheartj/ehy136.

221. Giustozzi, M. *et al.* Concomitant use of direct oral anticoagulants and antiepileptic drugs: a prospective cohort study in patients with atrial fibrillation. *Clin Drug Investig* 2021; 41: 43–51, doi:10.1007/s40261-020-00982-8.

222. Gronich, N., Stein, N. & Muszkat, M. Association between use of pharmacokinetic-interacting drugs and effectiveness and safety of direct acting oral anticoagulants: nested case-control study. *Clin Pharmacol Ther* 2021; 110: 1526–1536, doi:10.1002/cpt.2369.

223. Candeloro, M. *et al.* Carbamazepine, phenytoin, and oral anticoagulants: Drug-drug interaction and clinical events in a retrospective cohort. *Res Pract Thromb Haemost* 2022; 6: e12650, doi:10.1002/rth2.12650.

224. Li, A. *et al.* Drug-drug interactions with direct oral anticoagulants associated with adverse events in the real world: A systematic review. *Thromb Res* 2020; 194: 240–245, doi:10.1016/j.thromres.2020.08.016.

225. Song, D. *et al.* Lithium attenuates blood-brain barrier damage and brain edema following intracerebral hemorrhage via an endothelial Wnt/β-catenin signaling-dependent mechanism in mice. *CNS Neurosci Ther* 2022; 28: 862–872, doi:10.1111/cns.13832.

226. Oguzoglu, A. S. *et al.* Pregabalin protects brain tissue from subarachnoid hemorrhage by enhancing HIF-1α/eNOS signaling and VEGF production. *World Neurosurg* 2021; 152: e713–e720, doi:10.1016/j.wneu.2021.06.011.

227. Cholongitas, E. *et al.* Recurrence of upper gastrointestinal bleeding after donepezil administration. *Alzheimer Dis Assoc Disord* 2006; 20: 326, doi:10.1097/01.wad.0000213851.59119.0b.

228. Kok, K. S. *et al.* Upper gastrointestinal bleed associated with cholinesterase inhibitor use. *BMJ Case Reports* 2015, doi:10.1136/bcr-2015-211859.

229. Gareri, P. *et al.* Melaena following Use of the Cholinesterase Inhibitor Rivastigmine. *Clinical Drug Investigation* 2005; 25: 215–217, doi:10.2165/00044011-200525030-00008.

230. Bennett, J. A. *et al.* Acetylcholine Inhibits Platelet Activation. *J Pharmacol Exp Ther* 2019; 369: 182–187, doi:10.1124/jpet.118.253583.

231. Thavorn, K. *et al.* Upper gastrointestinal bleeding in elderly adults with dementia receiving cholinesterase inhibitors: a population-based cohort study. *J Am Geriatr Soc* 2014; 62: 382–384, doi:10.1111/jgs.12670.

232. Nissen, S. E. ADHD Drugs and Cardiovascular Risk. *N Engl J Med* 2006; 354: 1445–1448, doi:10.1056/NEJMp068049.

233. Winterstein, A. G. *et al.* Cardiac Safety of Central Nervous System Stimulants in Children and Adolescents With Attention-Deficit/Hyperactivity Disorder. *Pediatrics* 2007; 120: e1494–e1501, doi:10.1542/peds.2007-0675.

234. Cooper, W. O. *et al.* ADHD drugs and serious cardiovascular events in children and young adults. *N Engl J Med* 2011; **365**: 1896–1904, doi:10.1056/NEJMoa1110212.

235. Habel, L. A. *et al.* ADHD medications and risk of serious cardiovascular events in young and middle-aged adults. *JAMA* 2011; **306**: 2673–2683, doi:10.1001/jama.2011.1830.

236. Shin, J.-Y. *et al.* Cardiovascular safety of methylphenidate among children and young people with attention-deficit/hyperactivity disorder (ADHD): nationwide self controlled case series study. *BMJ* 2016; **353**: i2550, doi:10.1136/bmj.i2550.

237. Li, L. *et al.* Attention-deficit/hyperactivity disorder as a risk factor for cardiovascular diseases: a nationwide population-based cohort study. *World Psychiatry* 2022; **21**: 452–459, doi:10.1002/wps.21020.

238. Schelleman, H. *et al.* Methylphenidate and risk of serious cardiovascular events in adults. *Am J Psychiatry* 2012; **169**: 178–185, doi:10.1176/appi.ajp.2011.11010125.

239. Holick, C. N. *et al.* Atomoxetine and cerebrovascular outcomes in adults. *J Clin Psychopharmacol* 2009; **29**: 453–460, doi:10.1097/JCP.0b013e3181b2b828.

240. Zhang, L. *et al.* Risk of cardiovascular diseases associated with medications used in attention-deficit/hyperactivity disorder: a systematic review and meta-analysis. *JAMA Netw Open* 2022; **5**: e2243597, doi:10.1001/jamanetworkopen.2022.43597.

241. Coghill, D. R. *et al.* A systematic review of the safety of lisdexamfetamine dimesylate. *CNS Drugs* 2014; **28**: 497–511, doi:10.1007/s40263-014-0166-2.

242. Forns, J. *et al.* Risk of major cardiovascular and cerebrovascular events in users of lisdexamfetamine and other medications for attention-deficit/hyperactivity disorder in Denmark and Sweden: a population-based cohort study. *Neurology and Therapy* 2022; **11**: 1659–1676, doi:10.1007/s40120-022-00396-y.

243. Tadrous, M. *et al.* Assessment of stimulant use and cardiovascular event risks among older adults. *JAMA Netw Open* **4**: e2130795, doi:10.1001/jamanetworkopen.2021.30795 (2021).

244. Jeong, H. E. *et al.* Association between methylphenidate and risk of myocardial infarction: a multinational self-controlled case series study. *Pharmacoepidemiol Drug Saf* 2021; **30**: 1458–1467, doi:10.1002/pds.5322.

245. Mick, E., McManus, D. D. & Goldberg, R. J. Meta-analysis of increased heart rate and blood pressure associated with CNS stimulant treatment of ADHD in adults. *Eur Neuropsychopharmacol* 2013; **23**: 534–541, doi:10.1016/j.euroneuro.2012.06.011.

246. Liang, E. F. *et al.* The effect of methylphenidate and atomoxetine on heart rate and systolic blood pressure in young people and adults with attention-deficit hyperactivity disorder (ADHD): Systematic review, meta-analysis, and meta-regression. *Int J Environ Res Public Health* 2018; **15**: doi:10.3390/ijerph15081789.

247. Topriceanu, C.-C., Moon, J. C., Captur, G. & Perera, B. The use of attention-deficit hyperactivity disorder medications in cardiac disease. *Front Neurosci* 2022; **16**: doi:10.3389/fnins.2022.1020961.

248. Tisdale, J. E. *et al.* Drug-induced arrhythmias: A scientific statement from the American Heart Association. *Circulation* 2020; **142**: e214–e233, doi:10.1161/cir.0000000000000905.

249. Kelly, A. S. *et al.* Cardiac autonomic dysfunction and arterial stiffness among children and adolescents with attention deficit hyperactivity disorder treated with stimulants. *J Pediatrics* 2014; **165**: 755–759, doi: https://doi.org/10.1016/j.jpeds.2014.05.043.

250. Curtis, B. M. & O'Keefe, J. H. Autonomic tone as a cardiovascular risk factor: the dangers of chronic fight or flight. *Mayo Clin Proceedings* 2002; **77**: 45–54, doi: https://doi.org/10.4065/77.1.45.

251. eMc. in *Electronic Medicines Compendium* (2016).

252. FDA. FDA Drug Product Label. (2023).

253. Hermann, D. J. *et al.* Comparison of verapamil, diltiazem, and labetalol on the bioavailability and metabolism of imipramine. *J Clin Pharmacol* 1992; **32**: 176–183, doi:10.1002/j.1552-4604.1992.tb03823.x.

254. Juurlink, D. N., Mamdani, M. M., Kopp, A., Herrmann, N. & Laupacis, A. A population-based assessment of the potential interaction between serotonin-specific reuptake inhibitors and digoxin. *Br J Clin Psych* 2005; **59**: doi:10.1111/j.1365-2125.2005.02230.x.

Chapter 2

Chronic Obstructive Pulmonary Disorder

CONTENTS

The Maudsley® Prescribing Guidelines for Mental Health Conditions in Physical Illness, First Edition.
Siobhan Gee and David M. Taylor.
© 2025 John Wiley & Sons Ltd. Published 2025 by John Wiley & Sons Ltd.

INTRODUCTION

Treatment of COPD

Chronic obstructive pulmonary disease (COPD) is a common, preventable, and treatable disease characterised by persistent respiratory symptoms. These include breathlessness, chronic cough or sputum production, and frequent chest infections. Airflow limitation is progressive and not fully reversible. The aim of treatment is to reduce symptom burden, minimise the risk and severity of exacerbations, and reduce mortality. It must always include smoking cessation support. Drug treatment should include short-acting beta-2 agonists (SABAs – salbutamol, terbutaline) or short-acting muscarinic antagonists (SAMAs – ipratropium), long-acting beta-2 agonists (LABAs – salmeterol, formoterol) and/or long-acting muscarinic antagonists (LAMAs – tiotropium). Particular patients may require inhaled corticosteroids (ICS – beclomethasone, budesonide, fluticasone furoate), methylxanthines (theophylline), mucolytics, prophylactic antibiotics (azithromycin), oral phosphodiesterase-4 inhibitors (roflumilast), or oral corticosteriods[1].

Mental illness in COPD

Depression and anxiety are common comorbidities in patients with COPD. Reported prevalence varies widely (depression, 8–80%; anxiety, 6–74%[2]), and there is a link to severity of illness – patients with severe COPD are twice as likely to develop depression compared to patients with mild illness, and depression and anxiety worsen COPD outcomes (including hospitalisation rates[3] and mortality[4]). Patients with depression and COPD who take antidepressants are more likely to adhere to their COPD treatment[5,6]. There are few high-quality trials examining the efficacy and safety of pharmacological treatments for depression or anxiety in patients with COPD[7,8], so medication choice is instead informed largely by data derived from the non-COPD population. It is worth noting that some symptoms of COPD are similar to those in anxiety and depression – notably fatigue, altered sleep, and weight loss – and this might make decisions about treatment effectiveness more difficult.

Patients with schizophrenia or bipolar disorder are more likely than their counterparts in the general population to suffer with COPD (odds ratios from meta-analyses of 1.573 and 1.551, respectively[9]), and proportions of undiagnosed illness may be high (1 in 4 smokers with serious mental illness (SMI) had undiagnosed COPD in one study[10]). The reason for this association is unlikely to be limited to the higher rates of smoking amongst patients with schizophrenia or bipolar disorder[11]; rather, poor self-care, social deprivation, and the prevalence of other physical comorbidities in people with SMI are considered important[9]. Unfortunately, there is also evidence to suggest inequalities in the quality of care after diagnosis, and for increased mortality following acute exacerbations of COPD for patients with schizophrenia compared to those without[12].

The concerns with treating mental illness in a person with COPD are primarily based on overlapping drug side-effect profiles (e.g. anticholinergic effects, respiratory depression, or propensity to cause arrhythmias), or direct pharmacokinetic interactions. Most of these are theoretical, and there are few absolute contraindications. If psychotropic treatment is warranted but options are limited by the current airways prescription, each respiratory therapy should be reviewed by the patient's lung clinician to determine its ongoing need and to consider alternatives that may pose less risk.

ANTIDEPRESSANTS IN COPD

As already noted, it is not clear whether antidepressant treatment for patients with depression and COPD is effective – data specifically relating to the COPD population are scarce and fraught with the confounders common to chronic medical illness. Even fewer data are available to compare drugs, or even just drug classes with each other. Small studies and case reports describe the use of selective serotonin reuptake inhibitors (SSRIs) and tricyclic antidepressants (TCAs) in patients with depression and COPD[13,14]. TCAs are not usually considered first-line treatment for depression in the non-COPD population, and for those with COPD, the potential for additive anticholinergic effects from muscarinic antagonist bronchodilators such as tiotropium and ipratropium will diminish their appeal further (although in practical terms, this is probably only theoretical; see section on drug interactions).

One large cohort study found a worsening of respiratory-related morbidity and mortality in patients with COPD who were new users of SSRIs and serotonin-noradrenaline reuptake inhibitors (SNRIs)[15]. This appears alarming but should prompt close monitoring (adverse event rates remained small) rather than contraindicating use. Moreover, as beta-2 agonists can lead to dose-related QT interval prolongation and hypokalaemia, the risk of serious arrhythmia is theoretically increased if patients are also taking other agents that may prolong the QT interval or cause other cardiac arrhythmias. This makes TCAs, citalopram, and escitalopram less sensible choices (see section on drug interactions).

Breathlessness

There may be a relationship between depression, anxiety, and breathlessness, with symptoms of anxiety and depression being linked to the development of dyspnoea[16]; thus, treating the concurrent mood disorder may ease respiratory symptoms. In addition, some authors have suggested a role for antidepressants specifically in the direct treatment of breathlessness via inhibition of fear responses, altering the patient's perception of, and emotional response to, unpleasant stimuli such as breathlessness[17]. Sertraline was not effective when examined in an RCT for this indication (although it did benefit quality of life)[18]. Mirtazapine appears theoretically promising but as yet unproven beyond case series[17].

Smoking cessation

Smoking cessation is of vital importance in the management of COPD, and COPD patients who continue to smoke are more likely to suffer depression[19]. The antidepressants bupropion and nortriptyline have both been used in smoking cessation, although they are not considered the most effective options (for COPD patients this is varenicline and combined NRT[20]). Nortriptyline showed benefits to depression and anxiety symptoms in a single small study in patients with COPD[21]. The efficacy of bupropion for the treatment of depression or anxiety in patients with COPD is unproven. Although treating psychiatric symptoms and enabling smoking cessation with one single drug is an attractive prospect, given the importance of stopping smoking in this population it is probably preferable to try the most effective treatment (varenicline) for this indication first, and treat the depression or anxiety separately. If other smoking cessation strategies have failed, then it might be reasonable to consider bupropion earlier in the treatment cascade for depression. Note also that bupropion is unlicensed for the treatment of depression in some countries.

If patients are already prescribed bupropion for smoking cessation but depressive symptoms persist, then combining bupropion with other antidepressants is possible. Bupropion was used as an augmenting agent to citalopram in the STAR*D trial[22], and is usually well tolerated, although it is known to lower the seizure threshold in a dose-dependent manner and inhibit CYP2D6. Cautious dosing of the added antidepressant is recommended.

Summary

Choose an SSRI (avoid citalopram and escitalopram), or mirtazapine if sleep disturbance or poor appetite are particular problems. Consider bupropion (not first line), especially if other smoking cessation strategies have failed.

ANXIOLYTICS IN COPD

Antidepressants are generally recommended first line for anxiety, but other anxiolytics or sedatives (benzodiazepines, promethazine, pregabalin) may also be prescribed.

Benzodiazepines

Prescribers often worry about the risk of benzodiazepines causing respiratory depression. The reality is that benzodiazepines rarely cause respiratory depression in patients without pre-existing respiratory compromise outside overdose or use with other potent respiratory depressants (e.g. significant alcohol use)[23]. For patients with COPD, the magnitude of risk associated with benzodiazepines is unclear. Benzodiazepines are used in patients with COPD to treat breathlessness, especially in end-stage disease.

Some small studies of acute administration of benzodiazepines (single dose or short course) reported reduction in pulmonary function in patients with COPD (decreased tidal volume and oxygen saturation, reduced ventilatory drive and respiratory muscle function)[24]. Population data on adverse events of low-dose benzodiazepines in patients with COPD are conflicting in their results[25]. Some find no increased rates of hospital admissions but small increases in mortality[26], others find increased rates of admission[27] and respiratory adverse events[28]. Severity of disease, age of the patient (older adults are at increased risk of medication-related adverse events), and concurrent prescriptions (other respiratory depressants such as opioids) may be important, although confounding may also skew results that suggest these as influential factors (benzodiazepines may be more likely to be prescribed in severe, end of life disease).

Other risks associated with benzodiazepines include confusion, falls, and pneumonia, and again these may be compounded by other co-prescribed drugs (opioids, for example). Overall, it seems prudent to refrain from benzodiazepine use as far as possible for all patients, especially those who are physically frail or who have multiple comorbidities, and this should probably be extended to patients with COPD. There may be circumstances under which the benefits (both physical and mental) from short-term, 'crisis' use of benzodiazepines may outweigh the risks (acute anxiety, for example).

Promethazine

Promethazine is an anticholinergic drug, and so (as for TCAs) may compound the anticholinergic effects of concomitant inhaled bronchodilators (but the risk is probably very small; see section on drug interactions). Like all antihistamines, it may also thicken bronchial secretions, making them more difficult to clear, so it carries a manufacturer's warning cautioning against use in patients with bronchitis or bronchiectasis. In practice, this is unlikely to be problematic, and indeed small studies suggest promethazine might improve exercise tolerance and reduce breathlessness in patients with severe chronic airway obstruction[29] or COPD[30] without altering lung function, possibly by reducing the feeling of breathlessness.

Pregabalin

Recently, concerns have been raised about the effect of pregabalin on the central nervous system, as a small number of cases of respiratory depression have been reported worldwide[31]. This appears to occur independent of other concurrent risk factors (opioid prescriptions, comorbidity)[32]. As a result, pregabalin should be used with caution for patients with respiratory disease. If possible, it should be avoided in patients with COPD and reserved for when other options are unsuitable. Patients who are also prescribed other CNS depressants, those who are older than 65 years, and those with renal impairment (which results in increased plasma concentrations of pregabalin) should receive lower doses.

Summary

Aim to use antidepressants first line in the treatment of anxiety. Promethazine is not recommended specifically for the treatment of anxiety or depression, but it may be a useful sedative agent. Avoid benzodiazepines and pregabalin if possible. Antipsychotics may be used, but see comments in the next section.

ANTIPSYCHOTICS IN COPD

Acute respiratory failure

Patients with COPD, as with all respiratory illnesses, are at heightened risk of developing acute, chronic, or acute-on-chronic respiratory failure[33]. Acute respiratory failure (ARF) occurring in patients with severe COPD may worsen pre-existing chronic respiratory failure, with the increased airway obstruction during the acute event putting an additional mechanical load on the already compromised system[33]. Avoiding any insults that may risk causing ARF, especially in a patient with COPD, is therefore wise.

A handful of case reports describe ARF in patients with COPD within the first two weeks of starting antipsychotics (typical, atypical, oral, and parenteral)[34], and these seem to be corroborated by an observational case-crossover study which found a 1.66-fold dose-dependent increased risk of ARF associated with antipsychotics[35]. Note that this finding has not yet been replicated in a trial, other than one nested case-control study from the same group showing a similarly increased risk in non-COPD patients[36].

It is suggested that the serotonergic, histaminergic, and dopaminergic effects of antipsychotics may impair respiratory muscle activity or cause central respiratory depression. Quetiapine in particular appears to have attracted several case reports describing respiratory failure after normal therapeutic doses used in delirium[37,38] and sleep apnoea[39]. These cases should not be taken to suggest that quetiapine is more likely to cause ARF than other antipsychotics; there is no obvious reason for quetiapine to be particularly problematic. Respiratory depression is reported in overdose[40], but this is also true for other antipsychotics. It is the antipsychotic of choice in some critical care units for treatment of symptoms in delirium, and so confounding by indication may be an explanation. Transient rises in plasma concentrations caused by reduced metabolism of quetiapine (e.g. due to hepatitis) may explain some of the findings in the case reports[37], and it is possible that there is additive toxicity in respiratory depression when it is combined with methadone or other opiates[41].

A further possible mechanism by which antipsychotics cause ARF is that of acute laryngeal dystonia (an extrapyramidal side effect) precipitating acute respiratory distress, and this has been described in the literature[42], including one fatality[43]. Finally, neuroleptic malignant syndrome may also cause acute respiratory failure[44,45].

The data published so far do not confirm causality and do not clearly show that any single antipsychotic drug or drug class is more or less likely to cause ARF than another. Given the published reports associated specifically with quetiapine, other antipsychotics should be used where possible, and quetiapine avoided. It would be prudent to dose antipsychotics extremely cautiously in people with COPD, especially in patients for whom metabolism of drugs may be compromised, given the association of raised plasma concentrations of antipsychotics with respiratory depression. Avoiding antipsychotics entirely in patients already experiencing acute respiratory failure would be wise if other pharmacotherapeutic options are available and/or if the benefits of antipsychotic treatment are unclear (e.g. in delirium[46]).

Infection

There is a somewhat complicated relationship between antipsychotics and the incidence of pneumonia. Many studies report an increased risk of pneumonia for patients taking antipsychotics (almost double compared with no use[47]), but not all analyses support these findings. Despite this uncertainty, it should probably be assumed that antipsychotics do increase the risk of pneumonia, including for patients with COPD[48]. The mechanism for direct causation is unknown. Sedation, dystonia, dyskinesia, xerostomia, hypersalivation, poor physical health, and impairment of immune response (especially for clozapine[49]) have all been suggested[50].

Where possible, use of antipsychotics should be minimised for patients with COPD, assuming that the risk of pneumonia (already heightened for patients with COPD[51,52]) is additive (although whether COPD is associated with increased mortality and morbidity from pneumonia has been a controversial topic[53,54]). It will, of course, be the case that for many patients with chronic psychiatric illness, long-term antipsychotic treatment is unavoidable. There is insufficient evidence to support choosing (or avoiding) any single drug over another (apart from clozapine, which does appear to be particularly associated with infections[49], but it is also a drug that cannot be readily replaced with another). Use minimally effective doses (some studies suggest a dose-related effect[55]), avoid polypharmacy (combinations of multiple antipsychotics and mood stabilisers may be worse[56,57]), and treat contributory side effects promptly (sedation, xerostomia, hypersalivation).

Be aware that plasma concentrations of clozapine may rise during periods of infection[58], and patients with chest infections who smoke may do so less frequently and/or with less efficiency, which also causes clozapine plasma concentrations to rise. Reduce doses by a third whilst awaiting guidance from plasma concentration monitoring for patients with severe infections (those that require hospitalisation), and for anyone with signs of clozapine toxicity.

Summary

Avoid use of antipsychotics for patients with COPD where possible, and especially where evidence to support benefit is limited (e.g. delirium) and/or other pharmacological treatments can be used (e.g. anxiety). Where use of an antipsychotic is essential, avoid quetiapine if possible. Be aware of the possibility of increased susceptibility to pneumonia for patients taking antipsychotics and minimise risks where possible. Reduce clozapine doses for patients with severe infections.

ADDICTIONS AND SUBSTANCE USE

Opiate substitute treatment

Respiratory depression is common in patients with opioid use disorder and may be undetected in routine practice[59]. The opioid agonists methadone and buprenorphine, just like opiates themselves, are respiratory depressants[59]. For patients with COPD, there may be an additive effect of these factors, increasing the risk of clinically significant severe respiratory depression in the event of any further respiratory assault (e.g. infection). In conjunction with their specialist addictions prescribers, patients taking methadone or buprenorphine should be encouraged to consider a reduction in dose to mitigate the risk of respiratory depression. Note that as a partial agonist, buprenorphine was thought to have less of an effect on respiratory drive than methadone, but recent data suggest this may not be the case[59].

Benzodiazepines

Individually, opiates and benzodiazepines increase the risk of adverse respiratory events in patients with COPD[28]. In combination, this risk is increased further[28]. Avoid prescribing in patients with opioid use disorders. If unavoidable, minimise doses.

Pregabalin

As discussed in the section on anxiolytics, pregabalin (and gabapentin) has been associated with respiratory depression. In patients who take opiates there appears to be an increased risk of overdose when heroin and pregabalin are taken together[60], and an increased risk of abuse of pregabalin as it also reportedly enhances the opioid high[61]. Avoid prescribing in patients with opioid use disorders.

DRUG INTERACTIONS

Beta-2 agonists

At high doses, particularly as nebulised therapy, SABAs can cause hypokalaemia. This increases the risk of torsade de pointes[62]. Prolongation of the QT interval also increases this risk. At therapeutic doses, most antidepressants do not cause QT prolongation, but some caution may be warranted with citalopram and escitalopram. While antipsychotics, particularly (but not limited to) amisulpride, haloperidol, and quetiapine, are more clearly a problem, this is likely related to plasma concentration. Regular ECGs will confirm the absence of QT prolongation, and these are especially important in patients who may be exposed to large doses of SABAs (as in COPD).

Muscarinic antagonists

In theory, combining anticholinergic drugs, such as promethazine, clozapine, or clomipramine (not an exhaustive list – use medichec.com to check anticholinergic burden scores for individual drugs), with ipratropium or tiotropium would worsen anticholinergic side effects, such as dry mouth, blurred vision, constipation, urinary retention, and cognitive impairment. Note especially the risk for patients taking clozapine, who are already at heightened risk of death from gastrointestinal hypomotility. Despite the likelihood of any significant problems occurring in patients taking inhaled anticholinergic bronchodilators being low, the person should be assessed for these side effects prior to initiation of more anticholinergic therapy.

Theophylline

At very high plasma concentrations, theophylline can cause hypokalaemia, so the same warnings regarding torsade de pointes and QT prolonging drugs described with beta-2 agonists also apply here. The CYP1A2 inhibitor fluvoxamine causes rapid and potentially toxic increases in theophylline plasma concentrations – doses of theophylline must be halved[62]. Theophylline can lower the seizure threshold – many psychotropics are also known to do so (e.g. clozapine and bupropion).

Some case reports and small studies suggest that theophylline can counteract the sedation from benzodiazepines. The mechanism for the observation is unclear; it may be that xanthines block adenosine receptors, which regulate neurotransmitter release, leading to a stimulant effect[62]. There are no data examining the consequence of this interaction on the anxiolytic effects of benzodiazepines.

Theophylline reduces lithium plasma concentrations by around 20–30%, presumably by affecting renal clearance. This is an interaction that can probably be managed with careful monitoring of lithium plasma concentrations. Prior to co-administration, the need for theophylline should be reviewed by the respiratory clinician and plasma concentrations measured.

Azithromycin

Macrolide antibiotics are known to potentially prolong the QT interval, and it is possible that azithromycin will have the same effect[62]. Be aware of the additive risk if combining with other QT prolonging drugs (antipsychotics, citalopram, escitalopram, lithium) and of the potential for other drugs for COPD to cause hypokalaemia and further add to the risk.

Roflumilast

Fluvoxamine increases the plasma concentration of roflumilast by inhibiting the activity of CYP1A2, and the concentration of its active metabolite by inhibiting CYP2C19. This may be beneficial (increased clinical activity of roflumilast), but monitor for increased side effects (nausea, diarrhoea, headache)[62]. Note also that roflumilast has been associated with an increased risk of psychiatric disorders (insomnia, anxiety, depression, suicidal ideation, and suicide), and it is not recommended by the manufacturer for patients with a history of depression with suicidal ideation or behaviour[63].

PATIENT INFORMATION

Asthma and Lung UK, 'Looking after your mental health': https://www.blf.org.uk/support-for-you/looking-after-your-mental-health

Patient information leaflet: https://www.blf.org.uk/sites/default/files/Looking_after_your_mental_health_v2.pdf

CHAPTER 2

References

1. National Institute for Health and Care Excellence. Chronic obstructive pulmonary disease in over 16s: diagnosis and management (NG115); 2018.

2. Yohannes, A. M. *et al*. Depression and anxiety in chronic heart failure and chronic obstructive pulmonary disease: prevalence, relevance, clinical implications and management principles. *International Journal of Geriatric Psychiatry* 2010.

3. Pooler, A. *et al*. Examining the relationship between anxiety and depression and exacerbations of COPD which result in hospital admission: A systematic review. *International Journal of COPD* 2014; 9, doi:10.2147/COPD.S53255.

4. Atlantis, E., *et al*. Bidirectional associations between clinically relevant depression or anxiety and COPD: A systematic review and meta-analysis. *Chest* 2013; 144, doi:10.1378/chest.12-1911.

5. Wei, Y. J., *et al*. The association of antidepressant treatment with COPD maintenance medication use and adherence in a comorbid Medicare population: A longitudinal cohort study. *International Journal of Geriatric Psychiatry* 2018; 33, doi:10.1002/gps.4772.

6. Volpato, E., *et al*. The relationship between anxiety, depression and treatment adherence in chronic obstructive pulmonary disease: A systematic review. *International Journal of COPD* 2021; 16, doi:10.2147/COPD.S313841.

7. Pollok, J., *et al*. Psychological therapies for the treatment of depression in chronic obstructive pulmonary disease. *Cochrane Database of Systematic Reviews* 2018.

8. Usmani, Z. A., *et al*. Pharmacological interventions for the treatment of anxiety disorders in chronic obstructive pulmonary disease. *Cochrane Database of Systematic Reviews* 2011, doi:10.1002/14651858.cd008483.pub2.

9. Zareifopoulos, N., *et al*. Prevalence of Comorbid Chronic Obstructive Pulmonary Disease in Individuals Suffering from Schizophrenia and Bipolar Disorder: A Systematic Review. *COPD* 2018; 15, 612–620, doi:10.1080/15412555.2019.1572730.

10. Jaen-Moreno, M. J., *et al*. Chronic obstructive pulmonary disease in severe mental illness: A timely diagnosis to advance the process of quitting smoking. *Eur Psychiatry* 2021; 64, e22–e22, doi:10.1192/j.eurpsy.2021.12.

11. Dickerson, F., S *et al*. Cigarette smoking among persons with schizophrenia or bipolar disorder in routine clinical settings, 1999–2011. *Psychiatr Serv* 2013; 64(1): 44–50, doi:10.1176/appi.ps.201200143.

12. Jørgensen, M., *et al*. Quality of care and clinical outcomes of chronic obstructive pulmonary disease in patients with schizophrenia. A Danish nationwide study. *International Journal for Quality in Health Care* 2018; 30(5): 351–357, doi:10.1093/intqhc/mzy014.

13. Fritzsche, A., *et al*. Effects of medical and psychological treatment of depression in patients with COPD – A review. *Respiratory Medicine* 2011; 105: 1422–1433.

14. Yohannes, A. M. *et al*. Depression and anxiety in patients with COPD. *European Respiratory Review* 2014; 23(133): 345–349. https://err.ersjournals.com/content/errev/23/133/345.full.pdf.

15. Vozoris, N. T., *et al*. Serotonergic antidepressant use and morbidity and mortality among older adults with COPD. *European Respiratory Journal* 2018; 52(1): doi:10.1183/13993003.00475-2018.

16. Neuman, A., *et al*. Dyspnea in relation to symptoms of anxiety and depression: A prospective population study. *Respiratory Medicine* 2006; 100(10): doi:10.1016/j.rmed.2006.01.016.

17. Lovell, N., *et al*. Mirtazapine for chronic breathlessness? A review of mechanistic insights and therapeutic potential. *Expert Review of Respiratory Medicine* 2019; 3 (2): 173–180.

18. Currow, D. C., *et al*. Sertraline in symptomatic chronic breathlessness: A double blind, randomised trial. *European Respiratory Journal* 2019; 53, doi:10.1183/13993003.01270-2018.

19. Vestergaard, J. H., *et al*. Depressive symptoms among patients with COPD according to smoking status: a Danish nationwide case–control study of 21 184 patients. *ERJ Open Research* 2020; 6, doi:10.1183/23120541.00036-2020.

20. Antoniu, S. A., *et al*. Pharmacological strategies for smoking cessation in patients with chronic obstructive pulmonary disease: a pragmatic review. *Expert Opinion on Pharmacotherapy* 2021; 22(7), 835–847. https://doi.org/10.1080/14656566.2020.1858796

21. Borson, S., *et al*. Improvement in mood, physical symptoms, and function with nortriptyline for depression in patients with chronic obstructive pulmonary disease. *Psychosomatics* 1992; 33(2), 190–201. https://doi.org/10.1016/S0033-3182(92)71995-1

22. Trivedi, M. H., *et al*. Evaluation of outcomes with citalopram for depression using measurement-based care in STAR*D: Implications for clinical practice. *American Journal of Psychiatry* 2006; 163(1): 28–40, doi:10.1176/appi.ajp.163.1.28.

23. Kang, M., *et al*. *Benzodiazepine Toxicity* StatPearls; 2021.

24. Roth, T. Hypnotic use for insomnia management in chronic obstructive pulmonary disorder. *Sleep Medicine* 2009; 10(1): 19–25.

25. Currow, D., *et al*. Regular, sustained-release morphine for chronic breathlessness: a multicentre, double-blind, randomised, placebo-controlled trial. *Thorax* 2020; 75(1): 50–56. https://doi.org/10.1136/thoraxjnl-2019-213681.

26. Ekström, M. P., *et al*. Safety of benzodiazepines and opioids in very severe respiratory disease: National prospective study. *BMJ (Online)* 2014; 348, doi:10.1136/bmj.g445.

27. Vozoris, N. T., *et al*. Benzodiazepine drug use and adverse respiratory outcomes among older adults with COPD. *The European Respiratory Journal* 2014; 44(2), 332–340. https://doi.org/10.1183/09031936.00008014

28. Baillargeon, J., *et al*. Association of opioid and benzodiazepine use with adverse respiratory events in older adults with chronic obstructive pulmonary disease. *Annals of the American Thoracic Society* 2019; 16(10): 1245–1251. https://doi.org/10.1513/AnnalsATS.201901-024OC

29. Woodcock, A. A., *et al*. Drug treatment of breathlessness: Contrasting effects of diazepam and promethazine in pink puffers. *British Medical Journal (Clinical research ed.)* 1981; 283, doi:10.1136/bmj.283.6287.343.

30. Light, R. W., *et al*. Effect of 30 mg of morphine alone or with promethazine or prochlorperazine on the exercise capacity of patients with COPD. *Chest* 1996; 109, doi:10.1378/chest.109.4.975.

31. Medicines and Healthcare Products Regulatory Agency. Pregabalin (Lyrica): reports of severe respiratory depression. *Drug Safety Update* 2021; 14, 2.

32. Evoy, K. E., *et al.* Abuse and misuse of pregabalin and gabapentin: A systematic review update. *Drugs* 2021; **81**(1): 125–156. https://doi.org/10.1007/s40265-020-01432-7.

33. Budweiser, S., *et al.* Treatment of respiratory failure in COPD. *Int J Chron Obstruct Pulmon Dis* 2008; **3**: 605–618, doi:10.2147/copd.s3814.

34. Wilson, H. *et al.* Antipsychotic drugs and the acute respiratory distress syndrome. *Br J Anaesth* 2007; **99**, 301–302, doi:10.1093/bja/aem195.

35. Wang, M. T., *et al.* Association between antipsychotic agents and risk of acute respiratory failure in patients with chronic obstructive pulmonary disease. *JAMA Psychiatry* 2017; **74**(3): 252–260. https://doi.org/10.1001/jamapsychiatry.2016.3793

36. Wang, M. T., *et al.* Use of antipsychotics and the risk of acute respiratory failure among adults: A disease risk score-matched nested case-control study. *British Journal of Clinical Pharmacology* 2020; **86**(11): 2204–2216. https://doi.org/10.1111/bcp.14321

37. Chia, P., *et al.* Cardiopulmonary arrest following a single 25 mg dose of quetiapine: a case report. *J Crit Care Med (Targu Mures)* 2020; **6**: 253–258, doi:10.2478/jccm-2020-0035.

38. Jabeen, S., *et al.* Acute respiratory failure with a single dose of quetiapine fumarate. *Ann Pharmacother* 2006; **40**: 559–562, doi:10.1345/aph.1G495.

39. Freudenmann, R. W., *et al.* Respiratory dysfunction in sleep apnea associated with quetiapine. *Pharmacopsychiatry* 2008; **41**: 119–121, doi:10.1055/s-2008-1058111.

40. Strachan, P. M. *et al.* Mental status change, myoclonus, electrocardiographic changes, and acute respiratory distress syndrome induced by quetiapine overdose. *Pharmacotherapy* 2006; **26**: 578–582, doi:10.1592/phco.26.4.578.

41. Andersen, F. D., *et al.* Quetiapine and other antipsychotics combined with opioids in legal autopsy cases: A random finding or cause of fatal outcome? *Basic Clin Pharmacol Toxicol* 2021; **128**: 66–79, doi:10.1111/bcpt.13480.

42. Hilpert, F., *et al.* [Acute respiratory failure during long-term treatment with neuroleptic drugs (author's transl)]. *Nouv Presse Med* 1980; **9**, 2897–2900.

43. Yagmur, F., *et al.* Acute respiratory distress due to antipsychotic drugs. *Pharmacopsychiatry* 2010; **43**: 118–119, doi:10.1055/s-0029-1242822.

44. Soriano, F. G., *et al.* Neuroleptic-induced acute respiratory distress syndrome. *Sao Paulo Med J* 2003; **121**: 121–124, doi:10.1590/s1516-31802003000300007.

45. Johnson, M. D., *et al.* Neuroleptic malignant syndrome presenting as adult respiratory distress syndrome and disseminated intravascular coagulation. *South Med J* 1988; **81**: 543–545, doi:10.1097/00007611-198804000-00038.

46. Torbic, H. *et al.* Antipsychotics, delirium, and acute respiratory distress syndrome: What is the link? *Pharmacotherapy* 2018; **38**: 462–469, doi:10.1002/phar.2093.

47. Dzahini, O., *et al.* Antipsychotic drug use and pneumonia: Systematic review and meta-analysis. *Journal of Psychopharmacology* 2018; **32**: 1167–1181.

48. Ferraris, A., *et al.* Antipsychotic Use and Bloodstream Infections Among Adult Patients With Chronic Obstructive Pulmonary Disease: A Cohort Study. *The Journal of clinical psychiatry* 2021; **82**(3): 20m13516.

49. Mace, S., *et al.* Incident infection during the first year of treatment – A comparison of clozapine and paliperidone palmitate long-acting injection. *Journal of psychopharmacology (Oxford, England)* 2022; **36**(2): 232–237.

50. Taylor, D. M., *et al.* The Maudsley® Prescribing Guidelines in Psychiatry, 14 ed. Wiley Blackwell; 2021.

51. Farr, B. M., *et al.* Risk factors for community-acquired pneumonia diagnosed upon hospital admission. *Respiratory Medicine* 2000; **94**, 954–963, doi: https://doi.org/10.1053/rmed.2000.0865.

52. Almirall, J., *et al.* A. Risk factors for community-acquired pneumonia in adults: a population-based case-control study. *Eur Respir J* 1999; **13**, 349–355, doi:10.1183/09031936.99.13234999.

53. Jiang, H. L., *et al.* Is COPD associated with increased mortality and morbidity in hospitalized pneumonia? A systematic review and meta-analysis. *Respirology* 2015; **20**(7): 1046–1054, doi:10.1111/resp.12597.

54. Yu, Y., *et al.* Pneumonia is associated with increased mortality in hospitalized COPD patients: A systematic review and meta-analysis. *Respiration* 2021; **100**: 64–76, doi:10.1159/000510615.

55. Huybrechts, *et al.* Comparative safety of antipsychotic medications in nursing home residents. *Journal of the American Geriatrics Society* 2012; **60**(3): 420–429. https://doi.org/10.1111/j.1532-5415.2011.03853.x

56. Yang, S. Y., *et al.* Antipsychotic drugs, mood stabilizers, and risk of pneumonia in bipolar disorder: a nationwide case-control study. *The Journal of clinical psychiatry* 2013; **74**(1), e79–e86. https://doi.org/10.4088/JCP.12m07938.

57. Cepaityte, D., *et al.* Exploring a safety signal of antipsychotic-associated pneumonia: A pharmacovigilance-pharmacodynamic study. *Schizophrenia bulletin* 2021; **47**(3): 672–681. https://doi.org/10.1093/schbul/sbaa163.

58. Clark, S. R., *et al.* Elevated clozapine levels associated with infection: A systematic review. *Schizophrenia Research*, 2018; **192**: 50–56. https://doi.org/10.1016/j.schres.2017.03.045

59. Tas, B., *et al.* Undetected Respiratory Depression in People with Opioid Use Disorder. *Drug and Alcohol Dependence* 2022; **234**: 109401. https://doi.org/10.1016/j.drugalcdep.2022.109401.

60. Lyndon, A., *et al.* Risk to heroin users of polydrug use of pregabalin or gabapentin. *Addiction (Abingdon, England)* 2017; **112**(9): 1580–1589. https://doi.org/10.1111/add.13843.

61. Baird, C. R., *et al.* Gabapentinoid abuse in order to potentiate the effect of methadone: a survey among substance misusers. *Eur Addict Res* 2014; **20**, 115–118, doi:10.1159/000355268.

62. Baxter K *et al.* (eds). *Stockey's Drug Interactions*; 2022. http://www.medicinescomplete.com.

63. Electronic Medicines Compendium. *Daxas (roflumilast) 250microgram tablets*; 2022, www.medicines.org.uk.

Depression in Inflammatory Bowel Disease

CONTENTS

The Maudsley® Prescribing Guidelines for Mental Health Conditions in Physical Illness, First Edition.
Siobhan Gee and David M. Taylor.
© 2025 John Wiley & Sons Ltd. Published 2025 by John Wiley & Sons Ltd.

INTRODUCTION

Treatment of inflammatory bowel disease

Inflammatory bowel disease describes two conditions: ulcerative colitis and Crohn's disease. Ulcerative colitis (UC) affects the colon, while Crohn's disease may affect any part of the gastrointestinal tract. Symptoms include pain, diarrhoea, weight loss, and tiredness. Patients may also suffer with anaemia, arthritis, uveitis, and jaundice secondary to primary sclerosing cholangitis.

Pharmacological treatments may include 5-ASAs (mesalazine, sulphasalazine), immunomodulators (azathioprine, mercaptopurine, methotrexate, tioguanine), biologics (infliximab, adalimumab, vedolizumab, ustekinumab, golimumab), steroids (prednisolone, budesonide, beclomethasone), or other medicines such as tofacifinib, ciclosporin, tacrolimus, iron supplements, vitamin D, calcium, vitamin B_{12}, and folate.

Treatment of depression in inflammatory bowel disease

Rates of depression in patients with IBD may be twice as high as in the general population[4]. The prevalence of anxiety and depression is higher in those with Crohn's disease than ulcerative colitis[5], and women are more likely to suffer than men[5]. Comorbid anxiety and depression in IBD are associated with worse IBD symptoms (prevalence of anxiety or depression is higher in patients with active IBD compared with inactive disease[5]) and poorer adherence to medication, as well as increased hospitalisation and reduced quality of life[6]. The presence of depression increases the risk of developing IBD[7]; treatment with antidepressants mitigates this risk[7].

Tumour necrosis factor-alpha (TNFα) is known to play a role in Crohn's disease. Research suggests that (in the absence of medical illness) levels of inflammatory markers are raised in depression, and that antidepressants may change the circulating levels of these cytokines[6]. Meta-analysis shows that SSRIs may be associated with a reduction in IL-6 and TNFα levels, with other antidepressants having no effect[8]. Data are conflicting, however, with subsequent articles demonstrating TNFα lowering properties of mirtazapine[9]. How this should be extrapolated to drug choice in patients with pathologically raised levels of inflammatory markers, as in IBD, is not yet clear. Single case studies describe resolution of the symptoms of Crohn's disease following treatment with phenelzine[10] or bupropion[11] – both drugs that are thought to reduce TNFα by reducing intracellular cAMP[12]. The hypothesis for this mechanism of action directly affecting the symptoms of IBD remains theoretical and is not explored in clinical trials, so should not yet form the basis of decisions to select one antidepressant over another.

Up to 30% of patients with IBD are prescribed antidepressants[4], which may be used to treat depression, anxiety, or the symptoms of the IBD itself. There are few high-quality randomised controlled trials of antidepressants in patients with IBD[13], so decisions on the treatment of depression in patients with IBD are largely based on efficacy and tolerability data from the non-IBD population. It should be noted that the biological symptoms of depression that are measured by standard depression rating scales may not appear to improve on addition of antidepressants due to overlap of these signs with ongoing symptoms of IBD (e.g. fatigue). Antidepressant choice should be made based on the likelihood of adverse effects that would worsen the symptoms of IBD and/or comorbid conditions, and the likelihood of drug interactions with medicines usually prescribed for IBD and/or comorbid conditions.

Aims of treatment

The purpose of using antidepressants to treat depression in patients with comorbid IBD is to provide relief of depressive symptoms, with minimal or no adverse impact on the symptoms of the IBD or interactions with the medications used to treat the IBD. This chapter does not specifically address the use of antidepressants to treat the symptoms of IBD in the absence of depression, although some principles of drug choice described here may still be relevant.

Toxicity in overdose

As well as higher rates of depression and anxiety[5], IBD is also associated with higher rates of mortality in suicide compared to the general population[15,16]. Antidepressants have different toxicity profiles if taken in overdose, and this might be a relevant consideration when selecting drugs for individual patients. MAOIs (excluding moclobemide) and TCAs (excluding lofepramine) are considered highly toxic in overdose, and venlafaxine moderately so[17]. Other drugs are comparatively less toxic, but clearly may become more problematic if co-ingested with other substances, or where comorbid physical health issues are present.

CHOICE OF ANTIDEPRESSANT

GI side effects

Serotonin is heavily involved in gastrointestinal motility[18]. All drugs that affect serotonin receptors or serotonin levels may therefore affect motility. Additionally, drugs that act on central 5-HT_3 receptors can cause nausea and vomiting. Up to half of patients taking SSRIs or SNRIs experience GI side effects (abdominal pain, diarrhoea, nausea, dyspepsia) in the first few days and weeks[19]. Most side effects of this nature are dose-related. Using the lowest therapeutic dose should always be the aim of treatment. The use of modified-release preparations may help reduce these side effects[20], although data supporting this strategy are not consistent[21]. The aim is to achieve lower peak plasma concentrations and little fluctuation in plasma concentration from minimal to maximal.

Table 3.1 summarises a large recent meta-analysis[22] comparing gastrointestinal side effects of antidepressants (TCAs were not included). Note that data were restricted to short-term trials; it is not uncommon for gastrointestinal side effects to lessen after the first few weeks. It should also be noted that other analyses do not produce exactly the

Table 3.1 Gastrointestinal side effects of antidepressants

Nausea and vomiting	Diarrhoea	Constipation
Duloxetine (4.33)	Sertraline (2.33)	Duloxetine (2.58)
Vortioxetine (4.28)	Fluvoxamine (2.29)	Venlafaxine (2.45)
Venlafaxine (3.52)	Escitalopram (1.91)	Sertraline (2.38)
Sertraline (2.78)	Citalopram (1.64)	Paroxetine (2.14)
Fluvoxamine (2.72)	Duloxetine (1.60)	Agomelatine (2.10)
Escitalopram (2.51)	Agomelatine (1.39)	Vortioxetine (1.59)
Paroxetine (2.11)	Paroxetine (1.35)	Bupropion (1.52)
Citalopram (1.85)	Fluoxetine (1.29)	Fluvoxamine (2.14)
Agomelatine (1.77)	Vortioxetine (1.23)	Mirtazapine (1.46)
Bupropion (1.52)	Venlafaxine (1.00)	Citalopram (1.39)
Fluoxetine (1.45)	Bupropion (0.88)	Escitalopram (1.28)
Mirtazapine (0.73)		Fluoxetine (1.00)

Odds ratios compared with placebo given in parentheses.
Shaded sections are drugs that did not differ from placebo.
Note: No data available for mirtazapine and rates of diarrhoea in short-term studies.

same ranking[23,24]. Antidepressant choice for individuals should be informed by previous response to medication, predominant gastrointestinal symptoms, the expected interaction of the pharmacology of the antidepressants with these factors, as well as population data from clinical trials such as those presented here.

Patients with nausea and vomiting

Mirtazapine exhibits antinausea properties due to 5-HT_3 antagonism. All other drugs that affect serotonin availability in the gastrointestinal tract and CNS are associated with nausea and vomiting; TCAs and MAOIs may be preferable to SSRIs and SNRIs for this reason[22]. This effect may also be dose dependent.

   Recommendation: mirtazapine.

Patients with diarrhoea

Tricyclic antidepressants slow gastrointestinal transit due to anticholinergic effects, so they may be of benefit to patients with diarrhoea. The tertiary amines (amitriptyline, imipramine) are more strongly anticholinergic than the secondary amines (desimipramine, nortriptyline), so have more marked constipating activity. SNRIs may also exert this effect, as may mirtazapine. Although not included in the meta-analysis above, other reviews report low comparative incidence of diarrhoea associated with mirtazapine (6.4%[24]). SSRIs increase gastric motility via serotonergic activity so are best avoided.

Agomelatine is associated with low rates of diarrhoea (comparable to placebo) in clinical trials and lacks serotonergic activity, so is unlikely to worsen diarrhoea (or benefit it).

Recommendation: TCA (consider amitriptyline or nortriptyline), venlafaxine, agomelatine, mirtazapine or bupropion. If SSRI is required, prefer paroxetine or fluoxetine, consider vortioxetine.

Patients with constipation

Constipation caused by antidepressants is secondary to their anticholinergic effects. Tricyclic antidepressants are therefore associated with higher incidence of constipation than other drugs and should be avoided. Paroxetine, mirtazapine and trazodone are also more anticholinergic than other options so should probably be avoided as first-line choices, although the meta-analysis referenced above found no difference in rates of constipation between mirtazapine and placebo. SSRIs may increase gastric and small bowel motility due to effects on serotonin receptors, so may be of benefit to those with constipation.

Recommendation: SSRI (not paroxetine or sertraline), mirtazapine (possibly reserve as a second-line option).

Pain

Antidepressants are used to treat chronic pain (especially neuropathic pain), usually in lower doses than those considered therapeutic for the treatment of depression (Table 3.2). Drugs that affect both the serotonin and noradrenaline monoamine systems appear to be more effective[25] – for this reason, TCAs and SNRIs are preferred. Of the TCAs, some authors suggest that the tertiary amines (amitriptyline and imipramine), which inhibit serotonin to a greater degree than their effect on noradrenaline, may be more effective than the secondary amines (nortriptyline), which exert more effect on noradrenaline[26], although this is not found consistently. TCAs and venlafaxine have a NNT for neuropathic pain of 3[27]. Imipramine lacks a good quality evidence base to support use – other options have greater supportive evidence[27]. NICE[28] recommend amitriptyline or duloxetine as antidepressants for the treatment of neuropathic pain, but note that venlafaxine can be used in specialist settings.

Table 3.2 Antidepressant doses for neuropathic pain and depression

	Dose for neuropathic pain	Minimum therapeutic dose for depression[17]
Amitriptyline	25–75mg/day[29]	75–125mg/day
Nortriptyline	10–75mg[30]	75–125mg/day
Duloxetine	60–120mg[26]	60mg/day
Venlafaxine	>150mg/day[26]	75mg/day

Note: unlicensed use of nortriptyline, duloxetine, and venlafaxine.

CHAPTER 3

For patients with comorbid pain and depression not currently taking an antidepressant, it is sensible to choose venlafaxine or duloxetine as these options can be used for both indications at similar doses. TCAs are usually well tolerated in the low doses used for pain relief[31] but their side effects (principally those related to anticholinergic effects) may make them difficult to tolerate for patients with pre-existing gastrointestinal disorders at doses required to also treat depressive symptoms.

If patients are taking duloxetine or venlafaxine for pain relief but still experiencing depressive symptoms, the first step should be to optimise dosing; where possible, doses should be increased as far as tolerated. If this is unsuccessful or not tolerated, switching to a different antidepressant is preferable (choice should be made based on patient preference, concurrent drugs and other comorbidities, and previous response to antidepressants). If the patient does not wish to discontinue the SNRI because it is helpful in providing pain relief, then combination antidepressant therapy may be necessary. The combination of mirtazapine with venlafaxine is supported by the STAR*D study and usually well tolerated[32], although there is a risk of serotonin syndrome. Combination with agomelatine is likely to be safe, but efficacy is not proven and limited to case reports[33]. Further options include augmentation with lithium, quetiapine, or aripiprazole[17].

Where patients are already taking low doses of TCAs for pain relief and do not wish to discontinue, a second antidepressant may need to be added in order to treat depression. Combining TCAs with SSRIs or SNRIs presents three problems. First, fluoxetine, paroxetine, and to a lesser extent sertraline, citalopram, escitalopram, venlafaxine, and duloxetine inhibit CYP2D6, which is involved in the metabolism of TCAs[34]. Second, additive antimuscarinic and cardiac side effects should be expected. Finally, there is an increased risk of serotonin syndrome. Agomelatine lacks the serotonergic, anticholinergic, and CYP-inhibiting properties of the other drugs and therefore presents no problems in combination with TCAs. Combining low-dose TCAs with mirtazapine is probably preferable to combining TCAs with SSRIs because it also lacks the risk of serotonin syndrome or CYP inhibition but is more anticholinergic than agomelatine. The combination of TCA with SSRI or SNRI should only be attempted if other, safer options have been ruled out and should be undertaken with caution. Patients must be aware of the signs of serotonin syndrome.

Fatigue

It is helpful to first consider the nature of the fatigue, specifically whether **insomnia** is a contributing factor. Agomelatine, a melatonin receptor agonist, improves sleep quality in patients with depression by mimicking the natural rhythm of melatonin release[35]. Mirtazapine reduces sleep latency and improves total sleep time and quality[35,36] due to histaminergic activity. The effect on histamine receptors predominates at lower doses (<7.5mg). Noradrenergic effects become more apparent at higher doses (minimum effective dose for depression is 30mg/day) and drowsiness is reduced (although this is disputed[37]). Trazodone has a hypnotic effect in low doses (25–100mg), inducing and maintaining sleep without causing daytime sleepiness due to its short half-life (3–6h)[38]. Higher doses are needed to treat depression (>150mg/day), which are likely to cause daytime drowsiness.

For patients who are **fatigued without insomnia**, antidepressants with lower risk of sedation should be selected. Mirtazapine and trazodone should be avoided (but bear in mind that the sedative effects of mirtazapine may dissipate at higher doses), as should duloxetine and TCAs – these agents have greater reports of fatigue and sleepiness than placebo[39]. SSRIs, venlafaxine, and agomelatine have a similar incidence of fatigue to placebo in clinical trials so are preferable[39]. Bupropion has a unique mechanism of action in depression, involving dopaminergic and noradrenergic activity. In practice, it has an alerting effect and may therefore be useful in patients struggling with significant fatigue. It is unlicensed for this indication in the UK.

Be aware that conditions such as anaemia, vitamin B_{12} deficiency, folate deficiency, and vitamin D deficiency frequently occur in patients with IBD, and may cause fatigue. These should be investigated and corrected accordingly.

Patients taking corticosteroids

Depression, along with other psychiatric symptoms (psychosis, mania), is reported by patients taking corticosteroids. Psychiatric side effects of corticosteroid treatment usually have a rapid onset (1–2 weeks) and the incidence is dose related[40]. The risk may be increased by other drugs or conditions that increase the circulating levels of corticosteroids (clarithromycin, hypoalbuminaemia[40]).

The first step in treatment of corticosteroid-induced depression must be, wherever possible, to reduce and/or stop the corticosteroid. Tapering should be slow. Psychiatric symptoms can be induced by withdrawal of corticosteroid, especially if this is rapid[40]. If the steroid cannot be withdrawn, pharmacological management of the depressive symptoms may be necessary. No controlled trials are available to guide drug choice. Choice of antidepressant should be based on the usual criteria (patient preference, concurrent medication, comorbidities, previous response). See chapter 10 for more details on management of psychiatric disorders in patients taking corticosteroids.

Patients taking long-term corticosteroid are at increased risk of bone mineral density loss and osteoporosis. Serotonergic drugs can increase the risk of osteopaenia[41,42]. The risk of fracture is higher in a patient with frequent falls, and is further increased by concurrent osteopaenia. Data are mostly available for older adults, and should be interpreted cautiously due to confounding by indication. In general, the effect of the antidepressant on the serotonergic system is the cause of the fracture risk, so SSRIs are best avoided in vulnerable patients[43]. MAOIs (moclobemide) and NaSSAs (mirtazapine) may be preferable, but data are lacking to confirm this.

Note that omeprazole interacts with citalopram and escitalopram, and pantoprazole with escitalopram, in both cases potentially increasing the plasma concentration of the antidepressant and increasing the risk of dose-dependent side effects, including prolonged QTc. Rabeprazole is preferred.

Nil by mouth

In general, if oral access for drug administration is not possible for a short period of time (**days**), omitting antidepressants is unlikely to present problems. The drug can usually be restarted at the previous dose after the break in treatment (but use lower doses

CHAPTER 3

if the patient's medical condition has changed and they are more vulnerable to side effects). If the treatment break is likely to be longer than this (**weeks**) or the patient shows signs of depressive relapse or antidepressant withdrawal, alternative options may need to be considered. If it is possible to take small volumes of liquid by mouth, citalopram drops may be used (20mg is contained in 8 drops, equivalent to 0.4ml).

Other antidepressant options that are easily available in the UK (although unlicensed and with efficacy data limited to case reports) are to give the liquid preparation of fluoxetine sublingually (20mg/5ml), crush amitriptyline tablets and allow them to be absorbed buccally, or use orodispersible mirtazapine for absorption in the buccal cavity[44]. There is no guarantee that any drug will be absorbed this way. Orodispersible preparations of drugs such as mirtazapine and olanzapine are not designed for buccal absorption – rather, the drug disperses into saliva, which must be swallowed, allowing gastrointestinal absorption. Drug suspensions, or crushed tablets, are very unlikely to be absorbed at all (solutions are better, but most psychotropics have very limited water solubility). Plasma levels can be taken although are of use more to confirm that some systemic absorption has taken place rather than to establish whether a therapeutic level has been achieved (what constitutes a therapeutic plasma level has not been agreed for most antidepressants and is likely to be different for individuals). For patients who have been receiving sublingual or buccal medication for a week or two with no response, it is reasonable to check the plasma level to establish whether non-response is due to lack of absorption or treatment failure.

A further option is to use intramuscular flupenthixol decanoate – this is an antipsychotic depot injection with antidepressant properties. When used at low doses (5–10mg/2weeks) it is well tolerated. Onset of action is not immediate – several weeks may be required to achieve therapeutic plasma levels. Asenapine, an atypical antipsychotic, lacks data to support use in unipolar depression (and is not licensed for this indication) but is effective in the treatment of depression in bipolar disorder. It has the significant advantage of being designed to be entirely absorbed in the buccal cavity.

There are several non-oral preparations of antidepressants that can be obtained but usually not without some delay. Transdermal selegiline is licensed in the USA and can be imported for use in the UK. Intravenous clomipramine is a European preparation that can also be obtained. Intravenous citalopram is an unlicensed preparation that can be requested directly from the manufacturer.

Finally, esketamine nasal spray may have a particularly useful role for patients who are unable to take oral medications. At the time of writing it had not been recommended for use in the NHS by NICE, although it is a licensed medication in the UK. There is a growing evidence base for the use of intravenous, subcutaneous, or sublingual ketamine for depression; this may be easier to obtain. See chapter 13 for more information on non-oral administration of psychiatric medicines.

Management of patients with a short bowel

Drug absorption in patients with gastrointestinal disease is affected by several factors, including gastric emptying and transit time, and the length of intestine available for absorption[30]. The latter is of particular importance. The small intestine (duodenum, jejunum, and ileum) is the most important site for drug absorption, and within this the upper portion (duodenum and jejunum) play the largest role[45]. Slowing the rate of gastric emptying reduces the rate of intestinal absorption[45] – administering medication on an empty stomach with water improves this process. Aqueous solutions are more rapidly absorbed than solid dosage forms or suspensions[45].

If patients have had a portion of their intestines removed, or for other reasons drug absorption is expected to be limited in some or all of the GI tract, concerns are often raised about whether antidepressants will be absorbed into the systemic circulation. Predicting the effect of these conditions on antidepressant absorption and efficacy is difficult, and will differ for each patient depending on the extent of the intestinal resection. Plasma concentrations may be useful in elucidating whether *any* absorption is occurring, but as previously stated the relationship between plasma level and effect is not well established for most antidepressants. If it is possible to take a plasma level before surgery this may be helpful for comparison.

In Table 3.3, plasma concentration ranges are given where they are available. Note that these should not be interpreted as evidence-based therapeutic ranges. In many cases they are simply plasma levels measured at steady state for licensed doses, and the table gives the broadest ranges of plasma concentrations provided in the literature. Reported ranges frequently vary widely between studies and between patients. Observation of the patient response and comparison to levels achieved during a period of effective symptom control is much more important.

Table 3.3 Plasma concentration ranges	
Drug	**Range (trough, mcg/L)**
Amitriptyline[17,46]	80–200
Nortriptyline[17,47]	50–170
Fluoxetine[46,48]	80–300
Imipramine[46,47]	175–350
Mirtazapine[49]	5–100
Sertraline[20,46,50-52]	10–50
Citalopram[46]	30–130
Escitalopram[46]	15–80
Clomipramine[53]	100–250
Moclobemide[46]	300–1000
Paroxetine[54]	20–120
Trazodone[46,55]	260–1500
Venlafaxine[56]	10–200
Trimipramine[46]	150–350
Mianserin[46]	15–70
Vortioxetine[57]	9–33

CHAPTER 3

Modified-release drug formulations should be avoided. Soluble, liquid, or uncoated formulations are preferred. Little is known about the exact site of absorption of antidepressants. There are no clinical trials of administration of antidepressants to patients with short bowels, and few case reports. In the absence of data to guide drug selection based on pharmacokinetics, the following principles of prescribing are recommended.

For patients already established on an antidepressant which has been effective, maintain this treatment at the pre-surgery dose, switching to a liquid preparation if possible and converting modified release preparations to the equivalent immediate release. Observe response (preferably over several weeks). If relapse occurs (or symptoms of antidepressant withdrawal emerge), then increase the dose to no more than the licensed maximum. This is preferably guided by comparing plasma concentrations to pre-surgery levels, but if these are not available, then a dose increase in their absence is reasonable. If no response is seen after a further 1–2 weeks, plasma levels are strongly recommended before any consideration of increasing the dose beyond the licensed maximum. If a plasma level at this stage shows lower levels than achieved on a previously effective dose, consideration may be made to increase the dose beyond the license with the aim of achieving the previously effective plasma concentration. If this is not effective (assess over 1–2 weeks), not possible, or not acceptable to the patient or prescriber, then the antidepressant should be switched. Switching to another drug with a similar pharmacological activity is rational if response was good to the pre-surgery antidepressant.

For patients not already taking an antidepressant, drug choice should be based on the usual factors (patient choice, comorbidities, concurrent medication, previous response to antidepressants) and availability of the chosen agent in liquid form. Dosing should be commenced as normal and response assessed over 2–4 weeks. If no response is observed, a plasma level is recommended to establish non-absorption versus non-response. If the plasma level is low, increase the dose to the licensed maximum. If no response is observed, the drug should be switched.

Drug interactions

Mirtazapine + immunosuppressants

Bone marrow depression (presenting as granulocytopaenia or agranulocytosis) has been reported rarely (0.1%[58]) during treatment with mirtazapine. It is usually reversible on treatment cessation, but has been fatal (more likely in those over 65)[29]. The combination of mirtazapine with other agents associated with bone marrow depression is not contraindicated and there are no published reports of adverse effects of the combination, but knowledge of the potential for an additive risk may be useful. Regular blood monitoring is recommended routinely for patients taking immunosuppressants.

Tofacitinib + CYP inhibitors

Tofacitinib requires dose adjustment when administered with potent inhibitors of CYP3A4, or with moderate inhibitors of CYP3A4 in combination with potent inhibitors of CYP2C19[29]. This affects fluvoxamine (CYP3A4 and 2C19 inhibitor) and fluoxetine (CYP3A4 inhibitor).

Ciclosporin/tacrolimus + CYP3A4 inhibitors

Inhibitors of CYP3A4 may increase plasma levels of ciclosporin and tacrolimus[29]. Theoretically, this may include fluvoxamine and (to a lesser extent) fluoxetine. There are small numbers of case reports describing this interaction for ciclosporin and a small case series demonstrating no change in ciclosporin levels with concurrent fluoxetine. Ciclosporin and tacrolimus plasma levels are measured regularly in practice. Ensuring this is done when starting, stopping, or altering doses of these antidepressants is recommended.

Tacrolimus + QT prolonging drugs

Tacrolimus has been associated with QT prolongation. Concurrent use with other agents that also increase the QT interval may increase the risk. This includes antidepressants. Periodic ECGs are recommended[58] and TCAs avoided if possible.

References

1. National Institute for Health and Care Excellence. Depression in adults: recognition and management. depression in adults: recognition and management *NICE Guidance 222*, 2022. https://www.nice.org.uk/guidance/ng222.
2. Taylor, DM, *et al*. *The Maudsley® Prescribing Guidelines in Psychiatry* 14th edn. Wiley Blackwell, 2021.
3. Trivedi, MH, *et al*. Evaluation of outcomes with citalopram for depression using measurement-based care in STAR*D: Implications for clinical practice. *Am J Psychiatry* 2006; **163**:28–40.
4. Limketkai, BN, *et al*. Adjuvant therapy with antidepressants for the management of inflammatory bowel disease. *Cochrane Database of System Rev* 2019; 2(2). doi:10.1002/14651858.cd012680.pub2.
5. Barberio, B, *et al*. Prevalence of symptoms of anxiety and depression in patients with inflammatory bowel disease: a systematic review and meta-analysis. *Lancet Gastroenterol Hepatol* 2021; 6.
6. Mikocka-Walus, A, *et al*. Antidepressants in inflammatory bowel disease. *Nat Rev Gastroenterol & Hepatol* 2020; **17**(3):184–192.
7. Frolkis, AD, *et al*. Depression increases the risk of inflammatory bowel disease, which may be mitigated by the use of antidepressants in the treatment of depression. *Gut* 2019; **68**(9):1606–1612.
8. Hannestad, J, *et al*. The effect of antidepressant medication treatment on serum levels of inflammatory cytokines: a meta-analysis. *Neuropsychopharmacology* 2011; 36.
9. Gupta, R., et al. Effect of mirtazapine treatment on serum levels of brain-derived neurotrophic factor and tumor necrosis factor-a in patients of major depressive disorder with severe depression. *Pharmacology* 2016; 97.
10. Kast, R. E. Crohn's disease remission with phenelzine treatment. *Gastroenterology* 1998; **115**(4):1034–1035.
11. Kast, RE, *et al*. Remission of Crohn's disease on bupropion. *Gastroenterology* 2021; **121**(5):1260–1261.
12. Mikocka-Walus, AA, *et al*. Antidepressants and inflammatory bowel disease: A systematic review. *CP & EMH* 2006; 2:24.
13. Macer, BJD, *et al*. Antidepressants in inflammatory bowel disease: A systematic review. *Inflammatory Bowel Diseases* 2017; 23.
14. Szegedi, A, *et al*. Early improvement in the first 2 weeks as a predictor of treatment outcome in patients with major depressive disorder. *J Clin Psychiatry* 2009; 70, 344–353.
15. Zhang, C, *et al*. Incidence of suicide in inflammatory bowel disease: a systematic review and meta-analysis. *J Canadian Assoc Gastroenterology* 2018; 1.
16. Kaser, A, *et al*. Inflammatory bowel disease and completed suicide in Danish adults. *Inflammatory Bowel Diseases* 2010; 28: 573–621.
17. Taylor, DM, *et al*. *The Maudsley® Prescribing Guidelines in Psychiatry* 14th edn. Wiley Blackwell, 2021.
18. Gershon, MD. 5-Hydroxytryptamine (serotonin) in the gastrointestinal tract. *Cur Opin Endocr, Diabetes Obesity* 2013; 20.
19. Uher, R, *et al*. Adverse reactions to antidepressants. *Br J Psychiatry* 2009; 195.
20. DeVane, CL. Immediate-release versus controlled-release formulations: pharmacokinetics of newer antidepressants in relation to nausea. *J Clin Psychiatry* 2003; 64: Suppl 18.
21. Nussbaumer, B, *et al*. Comparative efficacy and risk of harms of immediate- versus extended-release second-generation antidepressants: a systematic review with network meta-analysis. *CNS Drugs* 2014; **28**(8):699–712.
22. Oliva, V, *et al*. Gastrointestinal side effects associated with antidepressant treatments in patients with major depressive disorder: A systematic review and meta-analysis. *Prog. Neuropsychopharmacol. Biol. Psychiatry* 2021; **109**:110266.
23. Kennedy, S.H, *et al*. Canadian Network for Mood and Anxiety Treatments (CANMAT) 2016 clinical guidelines for the management of adults with major depressive disorder: Section 3. Pharmacological Treatments. *Can J Psychiatry* 2016; **61**(9):540–560.
24. Gartlehner, G., *et al*. Drug Class Review: Second-Generation Antidepressants: Final Update 5 Report. *Drug Class Reviews* 2011; 1.
25. Jann, MW, *et al*. Antidepressant agents for the treatment of chronic pain and depression. *Pharmacotherapy* 2007; **27**(11):1571–1587.

CHAPTER 3

26. Sansone, RA, *et al.* Pain, pain, go away: antidepressants and pain management. *Psychiatry (Edgmont (Pa: Township))* 2008; **5**.

27. Saarto, T, *et al.* Antidepressants for neuropathic pain: A Cochrane review. *J Neurology, Neurosurgery and Psychiatry* 2010; **81**(12):1372–1373.

28. National Institute for Health Care and Excellence. Neuropathic pain in adults: pharmacological management in non-specialist settings. *NICE Guideline*; 2013.

29. eMC. Electronic Medicines Compendium. *Electronic Medicines Compendium*; 2016.

30. BNF. BNF 80 (British National Formulary); September 2020.

31. Riediger, C, *et al.* Adverse effects of antidepressants for chronic pain: A systematic review and meta-analysis. *Frontiers in Neurology* 2017; **8**:307.

32. Sinyor, M, *et al.* The sequenced treatment alternatives to relieve depression (STAR*D) trial: a review. *Can J Psychiatry* 2010; **55**.

33. Potměšil, P. What combinations of agomelatine with other antidepressants could be successful during the treatment of major depressive disorder or anxiety disorders in clinical practice? *Ther Adv Psychopharmacol* 2019; **9**.

34. Stockley, I.H. *Stockley's Drug Interactions*. Pharmaceutical Press, 2008.

35. Mi, WF, *et al.* Effects of agomelatine and mirtazapine on sleep disturbances in major depressive disorder: evidence from polysomnographic and resting-state functional connectivity analyses. *Sleep* 2020; **43**(11):zsaa092.

36. Dolder, CR, *et al.* The effects of mirtazapine on sleep in patients with major depressive disorder. *Ann Clin Psychiatry* 2012; **24**(3):215–224.

37. Shuman, M., *et al.* Relationship between mirtazapine dose and incidence of adrenergic side effects: An exploratory analysis. *Ment Health Clinician* 2019; **9**(1):41–47.

38. Jaffer, KY, *et al.* Trazodone for insomnia: A systematic review. *Innov Clin Neurosci* 2017; **14**(7–8):24–34.

39. Baldwin, DS. *et al.* Symptoms of fatigue and sleepiness in major depressive disorder. *J Clin Psychiatry* 2006; **67**.

40. Kenna, HA, *et al.* Psychiatric complications of treatment with corticosteroids: Review with case report. *Psych Clin Neurosci* 2011; **65**.

41. Wang, CY, *et al.* Serotonergic antidepressant use and the risk of fracture: a population-based nested case–control study. *Osteoporosis Int* 2016; **27**(1):57–63.

42. Rabenda, V, *et al.* Relationship between use of antidepressants and risk of fractures: A meta-analysis. *Osteoporosis Int* 2013; **24**.

43. Vestergaard, P, *et al.* Selective serotonin reuptake inhibitors and other antidepressants and risk of fracture. *Calcif Tissue Int* 2008; **82**(2):92–101.

44. Das, A, *et al.* Options when anti-depressants cannot be used in conventional ways. Clinical case and review of literature. *Person Med Psychiatry* 2019; 15–16.

45. Severijnen, R, *et al.* Enteral drug absorption in patients with short small bowel: A review. *Clin Pharmacol* 2004; **43**.

46. Baumann, P, *et al.* The AGNP-TDM expert group consensus guidelines: focus on therapeutic monitoring of antidepressants. *Dialogues in Clinical Neuroscience* 2005; **37**(6):243–265.

47. Perry, PJ, *et al.* Tricyclic antidepressant concentrations in plasma: an estimate of their sensitivity and specificity as a predictor of response. *J Clin Psychopharmacol* 1994; **14**(4):230–240.

48. Preskorn, SH, *et al.* Antidepressant response and plasma concentrations of fluoxetine. *Ann Clin Psychiatry* 1991; **3**.

49. Timmer, CJ, *et al.* Clinical pharmacokinetics of mirtazapine. *Clin Pharmacokinetics* 2000; **38**(6):461–474.

50. Mauri, MC, *et al.* Long-term efficacy and therapeutic drug monitoring of sertraline in major depression. *Hum Psychopharmacol* 18(5):385–388.

51. Warrington, SJ. Clinical implications of the pharmacology of sertraline. *Int Clin Psychopharmacol* 1991; **6**(Suppl 2):11–21.

52. Lundmark, J, *et al.* Therapeutic drug monitoring of sertraline: variability factors as displayed in a clinical setting. *Ther Drug Monit* 2000; **22**(4):446–454.

53. Stern, RS, *et al.* Clomipramine and exposure for compulsive rituals: II. Plasma levels, side effects and outcome. *Br J Psychiatry* 1980; **136**:161–166.

54. Tomita, T, *et al.* Therapeutic reference range for plasma concentrations of paroxetine in patients with major depressive disorders. *Ther Drug Monit* 2014; **36**(4):480–485.

55. Mihara, K, *et al.* Relationship between plasma concentrations of trazodone and its active metabolite, m-chlorophenylpiperazine, and its clinical effect in depressed patients. *Ther Drug Monit* 2002; **24**(4):563–566.

56. Charlier, C, *et al.* Venlafaxine: The relationship between dose, plasma concentration and clinical response in depressive patients. *J Psychopharmacol* 2002; **16**(4):369–372.

57. Chen, G, *et al.* Vortioxetine: Clinical Pharmacokinetics and Drug Interactions. *Clin Pharmacokinetics* 2018; **57**(6):673–686.

58. Micromedex®. IBM Micromedex. *Micromedex®* vol. V. 2.0; 2020.

Chapter 4

Critical Care

CONTENTS

DISCONTINUING OR CONTINUING PRE-EXISTING PSYCHIATRIC MEDICATION

A patient's regular psychiatric medicines (antidepressants, antipsychotics, mood stabilisers) are often stopped during an admission into critical care for various reasons, although the most common is the inability to administer medication by the oral/enteral route, which occurs when a patient is severely unwell. Routine cessation of antidepressants is not uncommon because of concern about continuing serotonergic medicines in patients who may be admitted with sodium imbalance or bleeding risks, or who require use of non-psychiatric serotonergic drugs (e.g. fentanyl). Cardiac instability may prompt worries about the effect of antipsychotics on the QT interval and the risk of QTc

The Maudsley® Prescribing Guidelines for Mental Health Conditions in Physical Illness, First Edition.
Siobhan Gee and David M. Taylor.
© 2025 John Wiley & Sons Ltd. Published 2025 by John Wiley & Sons Ltd.

prolongation, especially with interacting medication (e.g. fluconazole)[1]. Some clinicians consciously choose to stop all 'non-essential' medicines during periods of critical illness. Unintentional cessation of medication, not limited to psychotropics, is also common[2]. There is growing consensus, especially among specialist critical care pharmacists, to restart long-term medication in the recovery phase of critical illness[3].

There are no formal guidelines and scarce published data to support or inform decisions about whether to stop or continue psychotropics. Most research that is available focusses on discontinuation of antidepressants. Advice on handling of antipsychotics, including long-acting injectable formulations, clozapine, or mood stabilisers such as lithium, is limited to expert opinion.

Discontinuing

Discontinuation of medicines may be essential in the short term, if the oral/enteral route is not available. This also reduces the risk of drug interactions and of drug toxicity that arises because of accumulation during critical illness due to altered pharmacokinetics[4].

However, three problems may arise if psychotropic medicines are stopped. First, withdrawal symptoms may emerge[5]. These effects are well known with chronic and acute use of benzodiazepines, but may also occur on cessation of antidepressants[6] and antipsychotics[7]. Second, changes in medication can precipitate delirium[8], and therefore it is possible that stopping chronic prescriptions for medicines that alter neurotransmitter balances will have a similar effect. Third, there is the obvious risk that the patient's mental illness may relapse, potentially contributing to difficulties in weaning from ventilation and sedation and complicating engagement in medical treatment and rehabilitation. Importantly, a number of medicines (in particular, clozapine[9] and lamotrigine[10]) cannot be rapidly restarted once stopped.

Continuing

Continuing psychotropic medication may be unsafe or unwise in some circumstances. Many antipsychotics, and some antidepressants, are associated with QTc prolongation to varying degrees[11]. Tricyclic antidepressants may cause cardiac arrhythmia[12]. Anticholinergic medicines (tricyclic antidepressants, clozapine, promethazine) can slow gastrointestinal motility and worsen constipation[13], and there is increasing evidence of their adverse effects on cognition[14] and the risk of delirium[15]. Furthermore, rises in anticholinergic burden may increase the risk of acute cardiovascular events - see chapter one for details. Serotonergic medicines (e.g. selective serotonin reuptake inhibitors (SSRI), serotonin-noradrenaline reuptake inhibitors (SNRIs), vortioxetine) reduce platelet adhesion, thereby increasing the risk of bleeding[16]. These drugs also contribute to the risk of developing serotonin syndrome, particularly where other serotonergic drugs are also prescribed[17] (Table 4.1). Antidepressants and antipsychotics are also associated, again to varying degrees, with syndrome of inappropriate antidiuretic hormone secretion, resulting in hyponatraemia[18] (usually in the elderly, and within the first 4 weeks of use[19]). Where medical issues such as these are present, or considered to be a risk to the patient, the relevant psychotropic medicines should usually be withheld. If they are not, this can confound the differential diagnosis, which is especially important in severe hyponatraemia.

Table 4.1 Drugs that increase intrasynaptic serotonin	
Psychiatric drugs	Antidepressants (except agomelatine), lithium
Opioid analgesics[21]	High risk: tramadol, pethidine Medium risk: fentanyl, oxycodone, methadone, tapentadol
Antimicrobials	Iproniazid, linezolid
Dyes	Methylene blue
Drugs of abuse	Amphetamines, MDMA, cocaine
Parkinson's disease	Selegiline, rasagiline, safinamide
Anti-obesity	Sibutramine
Migraine	Triptans
Antiemetics	Metoclopramide
Antihistamines	Chlorpheniramine, dextromethorphan

Serotonergic non-psychiatric drugs

'Serotonin syndrome' is the excessive activation of peripheral and central postsynaptic $5HT_{2A}$ receptors, and a predictable result of excess serotonin agonism[20]. It is therefore not really a syndrome, but a form of poisoning. It is rare, and data describing relative prevalence with various drugs are limited to pharmacovigilance studies, so should be interpreted with caution. Where it occurs, it is most often the result of a combination of a psychotropic drug (usually an antidepressant) with a non-psychiatric drug[17]. Contrary to nomenclature, it is not just the SSRIs and SNRIs that affect serotonin. Various mechanisms beyond inhibition of serotonin uptake (as observed with SSRIs, SNRIs, TCAs, metoclopramide and antihistamines[21]) explain the increase in intrasynaptic serotonin caused by some medicines (Table 4.1). These include an increase in serotonin synthesis (e.g. tryptophan), inhibition of serotonin metabolism (e.g. MAOIs), increase in serotonin release (e.g. amphetamines), and direct activation of serotonin receptors (e.g. buspirone, triptans). The opioids (particularly fentanyl, tramadol, and pethidine, but rarely morphine and other related drugs), MDMA, and cocaine inhibit the serotonin transporter in a similar way to the antidepressants[21]. MAOIs relevant in critical care include methylene blue[22] and linezolid[23], others are iproniazid[24], selegiline, rasagiline, and safinamide (selegiline is licensed to treat depression in the USA). The anti-obesity agent sibutramine is an SNRI (although withdrawn from the market in many regions worldwide). Clinicians should also be aware of the potential for drug interactions in the context of hepatic or renal dysfunction that could further increase plasma concentrations of some medicines. This further increases the risk of serotonin syndrome.

It is unfortunately impossible to predict with certainty which patients will be able to tolerate combinations of serotonergic drugs and which patients will not. Consideration in each case should start with examination of the indication for prescribing each drug and whether a less serotonergic equivalent can be chosen instead. Where defined short courses of a drug are deemed essential (e.g. linezolid), withholding the other serotonergic drugs (usually an antidepressant) for this period is recommended.

Depots and long-acting injections

Some antipsychotic drugs are given intramuscularly in depot or long-acting injectable forms. Once administered, the drug cannot be removed. In critically ill patients, there may be a risk that the physical health of the patient will deteriorate (e.g. cardiac function deteriorates), or the capacity of the patient to metabolise and/or excrete the drug will change, (therefore causing accumulation of the medicine and potentially toxic plasma concentrations). In these clinical scenarios, use of these long-acting injectable forms of medication is inadvisable. Clinicians should be aware that plasma concentrations of long-acting injectable and depot preparations will remain present for weeks or months after the last dose was given. This means that administering missed doses is unlikely to be urgent (therapeutic concentrations may still be present) but, on the other hand, that side effects and toxicity may persist, despite apparent treatment gaps.

In general, it is usually better to avoid giving depot or long-acting injectable medication during periods of critical illness. Using an equivalent oral antipsychotic if required allows adjustment of doses in response to changes in pharmacokinetic handling of the drug.

Drugs with a narrow therapeutic window

The impact of critical illness on plasma concentrations of drugs with a narrow therapeutic window, including clozapine and lithium, is not well defined and thus unpredictable.

Lithium

Lithium plasma concentrations are affected by changes in renal function and renal perfusion, dehydration, and hyponatraemia[26]. Plasma concentrations must be monitored and doses adjusted accordingly.

Clozapine

Systemic infection may reduce the metabolism of clozapine via downregulation of CYP1A2 liver enzymes[27]. Stopping smoking has the same effect (olanzapine can also be affected)[28]. Monitor plasma concentrations and adjust doses as required.

Stopping clozapine can cause particular problems. Clozapine is uniquely effective, and it cannot be replaced with an alternative antipsychotic. Once treatment breaks extend beyond 48h, doses must be retitrated, a process that can take weeks. In the interim, patients are left without therapeutic plasma concentrations of antipsychotic, and relapse may occur. Safely managing symptoms of psychosis in a critical care environment can be extremely challenging. Clinicians may add a second antipsychotic to cover this retitration period (potentially compounding side effects such as QTc prolongation) but this strategy is unlikely to be particularly effective. Other sedative drugs may be required, or even complete sedation of the patient during the titration period, a situation that is unwelcome for patient and clinical team alike. Continuation of clozapine wherever possible is therefore strongly encouraged, utilising non-oral routes and formulations if required[29,30].

Restarting

There are no high-quality studies or randomised controlled trials examining the benefits or harms of continuing or discontinuing pre-existing psychotropic medications in patients who are admitted to critical care units. Where cohort studies, case series, and case reports exist, few report in detail the impact of stopping or continuing medication on mental health. Single-centre cohort studies have shown that restarting antidepressants earlier may reduce the incidence of delirium, result in fewer ventilator days, more time spent with the Richmond Agitation-Sedation Scale (RASS) score in acceptable limits, and a shorter length of stay[31,32]. Having a history of depression increases the likelihood of readmission to intensive care within a year of the initial presentation[33], and chronic mental illness is associated with worse health outcomes in a wide variety of medical conditions[34].

Withholding psychotropics during acute periods of critical illness may be necessary before the patient is stabilised and the oral enteral route is not available, but reinstating them as soon as practicable, and preferably before discharge from the intensive care unit, may improve both short- and long-term outcomes.

Note in particular the enhanced risk of relapse for patients who do not receive their expected number of depot antipsychotic injections over the course of a year (for example, where doses are repeatedly delayed or missed)[35]. If doses are delayed, subsequent doses must be given at the originally scheduled time (check individual manufacturer's guidance for details).

AGITATION AND ANXIETY

Agitation in patients on critical care units may have many causes, including delirium, pain, fear, and relapse of a pre-existing psychiatric disorder. This makes it difficult to wean patients from mechanical ventilation and/or from intravenous sedation, delaying liberation from ICU and increasing mortality[36]. It is beyond the scope of this chapter to discuss in detail intravenous sedation and agitation guidelines, but there is moderate certainty of evidence that dexmedetomidine may be beneficial for patients who are difficult to wean due to agitation, anxiety, or delirium[37].

For patients with known psychiatric illness, a first step should be to review any changes made to their usual psychotropic medicines. Consider whether agitation could be a result of withdrawal symptoms (e.g. has an antidepressant been stopped)? or relapse (e.g. have doses been omitted or reduced)?. If a patient usually smokes, consider nicotine replacement therapy. Restarting previous prescriptions (assuming they were effective) should usually be attempted first, before adding other medicines to treat acute symptoms.

Options for further pharmacological management of anxiety or agitation are benzo-diazepines, antidepressants, antipsychotics, and anxiolytics such as pregabalin. Benzodiazepines are effective in short-term, crisis use, but if the goal is to wean the patient from sedation, then adding further sedative drugs such as benzodiazepines can feel like a backwards step. Furthermore, lorazepam, midazolam, or high doses of any benzodiazepine are reported as independent risk factors for transition to delirium in critical illness[38]. A cohort study[38] showed the probability of transitioning to delirium for ICU patients increasing with lorazepam dose, with a large incremental risk at doses up to 20mg/24h (after which development of delirium became a certainty). Single, occa-sional doses of lorazepam may be less problematic, but if repeated doses are required it may be prudent to switch to a benzodiazepine with active metabolites (diazepam, clon-azepam). The longer effective half-life has been suggested to cause fewer problems with withdrawal, and possibly delirium (although this is still undoubtedly a risk). Buspirone is not recommended due to a long delay for the onset of action[39].

Antidepressants are usually considered first-line treatment for anxiety disorders, but the temporary increase in anxiety that often accompanies SSRI and SNRI initiation makes them less attractive for situations where controlling symptoms as quickly as pos-sible is imperative. Antipsychotics (particularly quetiapine) can be useful here. Pregabalin is also effective, although evidence in critical illness is lacking. Sodium valproate may reduce agitation and possibly delirium in this cohort[40,41] (aim for doses of up to 20mg/kg), but be aware that hyperammonaemia and thrombocytopaenia are common (19% and 13% of patients, respectively, in one study[42]). Additionally, critically ill patients may have lower albumin levels, resulting in a proportionally higher free-fraction of val-proate and a higher risk of adverse events. That said, the impact of hypoalbuminemia on drug pharmacokinetic and pharmacodynamics in critical illness remains uncertain[4]. Avoid promethazine (highly anticholinergic medicines may precipitate delirium, espe-cially when used with other agents which also have a high anticholinergic burden, including opioids and some antipsychotics, such as olanzapine[43]). Discontinuing medi-cations started for temporary anxiety states prior to discharge is recommended[44]. If rapid cessation is not feasible, then a weaning plan is essential[45].

SUMMARY

The appropriateness of continuing or stopping any medicine differs between patients, and in critical illness on a daily dynamic process depending on the patient's pathophysi-ology, including their end organ function[1]. In general, avoid discontinuing psychotropic medicines, including during periods of sedation, unless it is critical to do so (e.g. in scenarios where the oral/enteral route is not available or patient safety is a concern). Removal of chronic psychotropic treatment may result in relapse of the psychiatric condition and contribute to the risk of delirium, complicating weaning from mechani-cal ventilation and intravenous sedation. It is preferable to avoid giving depot injections to patients during periods of serious medical instability – use equivalent oral prepara-tions instead if antipsychotic treatment is required. Use plasma concentrations to guide dosing of drugs with a narrow therapeutic window (clozapine, lithium). Take into account pre-existing psychotropic prescriptions when considering prescribing for agitation and delirium agitation. Restart or optimise existing prescriptions in preference to starting new psychotropics. Consider restarting regular psychotropic medicines prior to discharge from critical care, and stop any that were started for temporary symptom control. If it is not possible to do so, ensure a plan for restarting/stopping is clearly communicated.

References

1. *Critical Illness*. 1 edn. Pharmaceutical Press; 2021.
2. Bell, C. M. *et al.* Association of ICU or hospital admission with unintentional discontinuation of medications for chronic diseases. *Jama* 2011; **306**: 840–847, doi:10.1001/jama.2011.1206.
3. Barrett, N. A., *et al.* Management of long-term hypothyroidism: a potential marker of quality of medicines reconciliation in the intensive care unit. *Int J Pharm Pract* 2012; **20**: 303–306, doi:10.1111/j.2042-7174.2012.00205.x.
4. Fraser Hanks, B. P., *et al.* How critical illness impacts drug pharmacokinetics and pharmacodynamics. *Pharm J* 2022; **308**: doi:10.1211/PJ.2022.1.126652.
5. Maffei, M. V., *et al.* Risk factors associated with opioid/benzodiazepine iatrogenic withdrawal syndrome in COVID-19 acute respiratory distress syndrome. *J Pharm Pract* 2022; 8971900221116178, doi:10.1177/08971900221116178.
6. Horowitz, M. A. *et al.* Tapering of SSRI treatment to mitigate withdrawal symptoms. *The Lancet Psychiatry* 2019; **6**: 538–546, https://doi.org/10.1016/S2215-0366(19)30032-X.
7. Brandt, L., *et al.* Antipsychotic withdrawal symptoms: a systematic review and meta-analysis. *Front Psychiatry* 2020; **11**: doi:10.3389/fpsyt.2020.569912.
8. Wilson, J. E. *et al.* Delirium. *Nat Rev Dis Primers* 2020; **6**, 90: doi:10.1038/s41572-020-00223-4).
9. Leyden Delta BV. Summary of Product Characteristics – Zaponex 25mg tablets. 2020.
10. GlaxoSmithKline UK. Summary of Product Characteristics – Lamictal tablets. 2022.
11. Funk, M. C. *et al.* QTc Prolongation and Psychotropic Medications. *Am J Psychiatry* 2020; **177**: 273–274, doi:10.1176/appi.ajp.2019.1760501.
12. Coupland, C. *et al.* Antidepressant use and risk of cardiovascular outcomes in people aged 20 to 64: Cohort study using primary care database. *BMJ (Online)* 2016; **352**: doi:10.1136/bmj.i1350.
13. Xu, Y. *et al.* Antipsychotic-induced constipation: a review of the pathogenesis, clinical diagnosis, and treatment. *CNS Drugs* 2021; **35**(12):1265–1274, doi:10.1007/s40263-021-00859-0.
14. Chew, M. L. *et al.* A model of anticholinergic activity of atypical antipsychotic medications. *Schizophr Res* 2006; **88**: 63–72, doi:10.1016/j.schres.2006.07.011.
15. Mueller, A. *et al.* Anticholinergic burden of long-term medication is an independent risk factor for the development of postoperative delirium: A clinical trial. *J Clin Anes* 2020; **61**: 109632.
16. Meijer, W. E. *et al.* Association of Risk of Abnormal Bleeding With Degree of Serotonin Reuptake Inhibition by Antidepressants. *Arch Int Med* 2004; **164**: 2367–2370, doi:10.1001/archinte.164.21.2367.
17. Pedavally, S. *et al.* Serotonin syndrome in the intensive care unit: clinical presentations and precipitating medications. *Neurocrit Care* 2014; **21**: 108–113, doi:10.1007/s12028-013-9914-2.
18. Seifert, J. *et al.* Psychotropic drug-induced hyponatremia: results from a drug surveillance program–an update. *J Neural Trans* 2021; **128**: 1249–1264, doi:10.1007/s00702-021-02369-1.
19. Mannheimer, B. *et al.* Time-dependent association between selective serotonin reuptake inhibitors and hospitalization due to hyponatremia. *J Psychopharmacol* 2021; **128**(8): 1249–1264. doi:10.1177/02698811211001082.
20. Boyer, E. W. *et al.* The Serotonin Syndrome. *NE J Med* 2005; **352**: 1112–1120, doi:10.1056/NEJMra041867.
21. Baldo, B. A. *et al.* The anaesthetist, opioid analgesic drugs, and serotonin toxicity: a mechanistic and clinical review. *Br J Anaesth* 2020; **124**: 44–62, doi:10.1016/j.bja.2019.08.010.
22. Ramsay, R. R. *et al.* Methylene blue and serotonin toxicity: inhibition of monoamine oxidase A (MAO A) confirms a theoretical prediction. *Br J Pharmacol* 2007; 152: 946–951, doi:10.1038/sj.bjp.0707430.
23. Antal, E. J. *et al.* A novel oxazolidinone antibiotic: assessment of monoamine oxidase inhibition using pressor response to oral tyramine. *J Clin Pharm* 2001; **41**: 552–562, https://doi.org/10.1177/00912700122010294.
24. Maxwell, R. A. et al. In Drug Discovery: A Casebook and Analysis (eds. Robert A. Maxwell & Shohreh B. Eckhardt), 143–154. Humana Press; 1990.
25. Heal, D. J. *et al.* Sibutramine: a novel anti-obesity drug. A review of the pharmacological evidence to differentiate it from d-amphetamine and d-fenfluramine. *Int J Obes Relat Metab Disord* 1998; **22** Suppl 1: S18–28; discussion S29.
26. Taylor, D. M. *et al. The Maudsley® Prescribing Guidelines in Psychiatry.* 14 ed. Wiley Blackwell; 2021.
27. Haack, M. J. *et al.* Toxic rise of clozapine plasma concentrations in relation to inflammation. *Eur Neuropsychopharmacol* 2003; **13**: 381–385, doi:10.1016/s0924-977x(03)00042-7.

28. Lowe, E. J. *et al*. Impact of tobacco smoking cessation on stable clozapine or olanzapine treatment. *Ann Pharmacother* **44**, 727–732, doi:10.1345/aph.1M398 (2010).

29. Gee, S. *et al*. Intramuscular clozapine in the acute medical hospital: experiences from a liaison psychiatry team. *SAGE Open Medical Case Reports* 2021; **9**: doi:10.1177/2050313X211004796.

30. Gee, S. *et al*. Alternative routes of administration of clozapine. *CNS Drugs* 2022; **36**: 105–111, doi:10.1007/s40263-022-00900-w.

31. Li, M. *et al*. Impact of early home psychotropic medication reinitiation on surrogate measures of intensive care unit delirium. *Ment Health Clin* 2019; **9**: 263–268, doi:10.9740/mhc.2019.07.263.

32. La, M. K. *et al*. Impact of restarting home neuropsychiatric medications on sedation outcomes in medical intensive care unit patients. *J Crit Care* 2018; **43**: 102–107, doi:10.1016/j.jcrc.2017.07.046.

33. Paratz, J., *et al*. Re-admission to intensive care: identification of risk factors. *Physiother Res Int* 2005; **10**: 154–163, doi:10.1002/pri.5.

34. Thornicroft, G. Physical health disparities and mental illness: the scandal of premature mortality. *Br J Psychiatry* 2011; **199**: 441–442, doi:10.1192/bjp.bp.111.092718.

35. Laing, E. *et al*. Relapse and frequency of injection of monthly paliperidone palmitate—A retrospective case–control study. *Eur Psychiatry* 2021; **64**: e11, doi:10.1192/j.eurpsy.2021.4.

36. Peñuelas, O., *et al*. Characteristics and outcomes of ventilated patients according to time to liberation from mechanical ventilation. *Am J Respir Crit Care Med* 2011; **184**: 430–437, doi:10.1164/rccm.201011-1887OC.

37. Dupuis, S., *et al*. A systematic review of interventions to facilitate extubation in patients difficult-to-wean due to delirium, agitation, or anxiety and a meta-analysis of the effect of dexmedetomidine. *Can J Anaesth* 2019; **66**: 318–327, doi:10.1007/s12630-018-01289-1.

38. Pandharipande, P. *et al*. Lorazepam is an independent risk factor for transitioning to delirium in intensive care unit patients. *Anesthesiology* 2006; **104**: 21–26, doi:10.1097/00000542-200601000-00005.

39. Goa, K. L. *et al*. Buspirone. A preliminary review of its pharmacological properties and therapeutic efficacy as an anxiolytic. *Drugs* 1986; **32**: 114–129, doi:10.2165/00003495-198632020-00002.

40. Quinn, N. J., *et al*. Prescribing practices of valproic acid for agitation and delirium in the intensive care unit. *Ann Pharmacother* 2021; **55**: 311–317, doi:10.1177/1060028020947173.

41. Crowley, K. E. *et al*. Valproic acid for the management of agitation and delirium in the intensive care setting: a retrospective analysis. *Clin Ther* 2020; **42**: e65–e73, doi:10.1016/j.clinthera.2020.02.007.

42. Gagnon, D. J. *et al*. Valproate for agitation in critically ill patients: A retrospective study. *J Crit Care* 2017; **37**: 119–125, doi:10.1016/j.jcrc.2016.09.006.

43. Clegg, A. *et al*. Which medications to avoid in people at risk of delirium: a systematic review. *Age Ageing* 2011; **40**: 23–29, doi:10.1093/ageing/afq140.

44. Alagiakrishnan, K. & Wiens, C. A. An approach to drug induced delirium in the elderly. *Postgrad Med J* 2004; **80**: 388–393, doi:10.1136/pgmj.2003.017236.

45. Devlin, J. W. *et al*. Long-term outcomes after delirium in the icu: addressing gaps in our knowledge. *Am J Respir Crit Care Med* 2021; **204**: 383–385, doi:10.1164/rccm.202104-0910ED.

CHAPTER 4

Surgery

CONTENTS

INTRODUCTION

Whether psychotropic medicines should be continued or withheld during the perioperative period depends on:

- physical status of the patient;
- the risk of the drug interacting with anaesthetic or perioperative medications;
- the likelihood of the drug contributing to complications in the perioperative period (e.g. CNS depression, delirium);

The Maudsley® Prescribing Guidelines for Mental Health Conditions in Physical Illness, First Edition.
Siobhan Gee and David M. Taylor.
© 2025 John Wiley & Sons Ltd. Published 2025 by John Wiley & Sons Ltd.

- the risk of withdrawal symptoms if the psychotropic is stopped, and the likelihood of these contributing to complications in the perioperative period (e.g. delirium);
- the risk of relapse of the underlying condition.

For the most part, psychotropic drugs should be continued during the perioperative period, assuming agreement of the anaesthetist concerned. Some anaesthetic and perioperative drugs are known to prolong the QT interval (e.g. desflurane, isoflurane, sevoflurane, domperidone, granisetron, ondansetron, ciprofloxacin, clarithromycin, erythromycin). Depending on individual risk, these drugs may be avoided, or, alternatively, ECG monitoring may be required for patients also taking psychotropic drugs that can prolong the QT interval. Other risks and benefits of continuing psychiatric medicines in the perioperative period are discussed in relation to individual drugs below.

ANTIDEPRESSANTS

SSRIs and SNRIs

Serotonergic drugs are associated with an increased risk of greater duration or severity of bleeding during and after surgery[1]. A meta-analysis of cohort studies found the bleeding risk may vary with the type of surgery, with orthopaedic procedures possibly conferring more risk[2]. Whilst stopping the antidepressant preoperatively would presumably reduce this risk, in practice this is not a simple task. Consideration needs to be made of the half-life of the antidepressant and presumed relationship between this time period and the effect on the platelet serotonin reuptake mechanism (responsible for the bleeding risk with antidepressants). Drugs with long half-lives – such as fluoxetine, for example – may need to be discontinued weeks, if not months, in advance. A further complication is that discontinuation symptoms are likely if serotonergic antidepressants are stopped abruptly, but recommended tapering periods are lengthy. There is also a risk of relapse of the mental illness during this period, which may jeopardise the planned surgery. Switching to an antidepressant with lower affinity for the platelet serotonin receptor may not entirely eliminate the bleeding risk, and there is a risk that that the new antidepressant may not be effective in treating the psychiatric illness. Withholding the antidepressant for only a few days around the time of the surgery is probably not rational, since there is no guarantee that platelet function will recover in this time, and the patient is then exposed to the risk of acute discontinuation symptoms.

Fluoxetine, paroxetine, and duloxetine are inhibitors of CYP2D6, the enzyme responsible for conversion of oxycodone, codeine, and hydrocodone to their active metabolites (oxymorphone, morphine, and hydromorphone, respectively). It is theoretically possible that concurrent use may result in suboptimal pain control. However, there is only a small amount of evidence for this in practice[3-5], whilst a larger number of studies find no clinical effect[6-9]. Consider using a different opioid analgesic that does not require conversion to active metabolites if necessary (e.g. morphine).

Several case studies report serotonin syndrome as a consequence of the combination of a serotonergic antidepressant and an opioid (including fentanyl, hydrocodone, hydromorphone, oxycodone, pentazocine, pethidine, tapentadol, and tramadol). Morphine does not affect 5-HT activity, so it is preferable[10]. Otherwise, patients who are given combinations of serotonergic drugs should be observed for signs of serotonin toxicity.

Some perioperative medicines (e.g. halogenated volatile anaesthetics, ondansetron, and metronidazole) may prolong the QT interval. The SSRIs citalopram and escitalopram may add to this risk[11], although as discussed in Chapter 1 on cardiac disease, the association between SSRIs and QT interval prolongation is disputed[12]. The inhibition of noradrenaline receptors by SNRIs increases both heart rate and risk of hypertension if catecholamines (e.g. ephedrine) are given during anaesthesia[13], although the effect in practice is unproven. It is possible that chronic use of SNRIs leads to physiological tolerance to these effects.

Abrupt cessation of SSRIs or SNRIs can result in discontinuation symptoms[14], which can be severe and may complicate diagnosis of postoperative symptoms. Furthermore, there is an increased risk of delirium when psychotropic medicines are discontinued in medically unwell patients[15,16].

Recommendation: SSRIs and SNRIs should usually be continued before, during, and after surgery. Anaesthetic agents and analgesics need to be chosen carefully.

TCAs

Tricyclic antidepressants are pro-arrhythmic owing to their shared ability to block cardiac sodium channels. They also antagonise cardiac noradrenaline receptors, and this sensitises the heart to further sympathetic activation, increasing cardiac output and blood pressure. The anticholinergic effect of TCAs may also contribute to increases in systolic blood pressure. The administration of sympathomimetic amines (particularly indirect-acting agents, such as ephedrine) during surgery to patients taking TCAs can therefore precipitate hypertension and arrhythmias[13]. However, as for SNRIs, the effect in practice is less clear, possibly because of the development of tolerance to these effects in chronic dosing of TCAs[13]. Guidelines from the European Society of Anaesthesiology recommend avoiding sympathomimetics in patients taking TCAs[17].

Amitriptyline and other TCAs inhibit CYP2D6 activity, so as described for some SSRIs and SNRIs, there is a theoretical loss of analgesic activity for some opioids.

Some guidelines suggest that enflurane should be avoided in patients taking TCAs because of the risk of precipitating seizures. This is based on a single report of two patients taking amitriptyline developing clonic movements during surgery when anaesthetised with enflurane, and the resolution of these movements when enflurane was switched to halothane[18].

As for other antidepressants, abrupt discontinuation of TCAs can result in withdrawal symptoms. Gradual tapering required to prevent such symptoms is unlikely to be practical preoperatively. Withholding the antidepressant for a few days around the surgery may avoid interactions with sympathomimetics but cause other problems. One

CHAPTER 5

study[19] of patients taking TCAs or mianserin undergoing orthopaedic surgery found an increased incidence of delirium or confusion in those who had their antidepressant stopped 72h before surgery. There was no difference in the incidence of hypotension or arrhythmias during anaesthesia for patients who stopped or continued the TCA.

Recommendation: TCAs can be continued perioperatively, but avoid giving indirect-acting sympathomimetics.

MAOIs

In the adrenergic neuron, noradrenaline is stored in two states – one bound to adenosine triphosphate (ATP) and one unbound and ready for immediate release. The enzyme monoamine oxidase (MAO) mediates the turnover of noradrenaline between bound and unbound states, thus controlling the amount of noradrenaline stored in the neuron and the amount available for release[20]. MAOIs form a complex with MAO, disabling it from performing this control function on noradrenaline stores. The amount of noradrenaline stored in the neuron increases. Indirectly acting sympathomimetic drugs (e.g. amphetamines, cocaine, ephedrine) release these stores, producing a potentially lethal hypertensive effect.

Opioids also interact with MAOIs. Two types of reaction can occur. One is 'excitatory', characterised by agitation, hyper- or hypotension, rigidity, seizures, and coma. This is thought to be due to serotonin overactivity[20]. The second is 'depressive', manifesting as respiratory depression, hypotension, and coma. This is thought to be due to inhibition of hepatic MAO[20], resulting in reduction of metabolism of the opioid and an increase in clinical effect. Of the opioids, pethidine is most clearly associated with the excitatory interaction, possibly because it is a weak serotonin reuptake inhibitor. Data showing this reaction in practice are limited to case reports. One prospective study that gave patients taking various MAOIs increasing doses of pethidine failed to provoke the reaction, implying that it may be a rare, idiosyncratic effect[21]. Other opioids with serotonergic effects include fentanyl, tramadol and tapentadol. A few cases of serotonin-like syndrome in patients taking MAOIs and fentanyl have been reported[22] (including one death[23]).

As a result of these concerns, the manufacturers of the irreversible MAOIs (tranylcypromine, phenelzine, isocarboxazid) contraindicate their use with sympathomimetic agents. They also recommend avoiding opioid analgesics due to the risk of CNS excitation or depression. Manufacturers' guidance is that patients taking MAOIs should not undergo surgery that requires general anaesthesia or be given local anaesthetics that contain a vasoconstrictor. They recommend discontinuation of the MAOI two weeks before surgery, but to avoid discontinuation symptoms this means beginning a tapering process long before this. Withdrawal of the antidepressant brings a risk of psychiatric relapse. Switching to a different antidepressant is also a lengthy process, as all switches require a 2- to 3-week 'wash-out' period once the MAOI has been stopped, before starting the new drug (other than agomelatine, which can be given concurrently)[24]. The choice of a replacement antidepressant may not be straightforward since MAOIs are frequently reserved as treatment options for patients who have failed to respond to other antidepressants. Another approach is to switch the irreversible MAOI to moclobemide, a reversible MAOI that can be held briefly to allow surgery or continued during surgery. This strategy still requires a 2-week wash-out period between cessation of the previous MAOI and commencing moclobemide.

There is some debate as to whether these strict contraindications are justified. One small retrospective cohort study found no difference in the occurrence of hypotension, hypertension, bradycardia, or tachycardia between users of moclobemide and tranylcypromine who underwent surgery[25], a finding echoed in other reports[26]. A consensus statement from the USA-based Society for Perioperative Assessment and Quality Improvement suggests that in practice, MAOIs are commonly continued perioperatively when 'MAOI-safe' anaesthesia is used (avoiding ephedrine, metaraminol, ketamine, pethidine, and suxamethonium)[17]. Other published recommendations concur with this stance[27]. It is clear that pethidine should be avoided entirely, as should fentanyl and tramadol, ideally. Morphine is safer as it does not block serotonergic transmission, but a CNS 'depressive' reaction is possible[28,29] perhaps in part due to the reduction in hepatic metabolism described above, so dosing should be cautious.

Recommendation: ideally, tranylcypromine, isocarboxazid, and phenelzine should be discontinued 2 weeks before surgery. If this is not possible or practical, they may be continued if 'MAOI-safe' anaesthesia is employed. Stop moclobemide the day before surgery (i.e. last dose to be taken 24h before surgery) and restart after surgery. If moclobemide is given on the day of surgery, MAOI-safe anaesthesia must be used.

Atypical antidepressants

Bupropion strongly inhibits CYP2D6 activity, so as described for some SSRIs and SNRIs, there is a theoretical loss of analgesic activity for some opioids. There are no significant perioperative interactions with mirtazapine or trazodone.

Recommendation: atypical antidepressants can be continued perioperatively.

ANTIPSYCHOTICS

Many drugs used perioperatively can prolong the QT interval, so ECG monitoring is recommended for most patients concurrently taking QT-prolonging antipsychotics (exceptions are lurasidone, cariprazine, brexpiprazole, and lumateperone). There is some evidence that patients taking antipsychotics may have impaired intraoperative temperature regulation owing to the effects of the drug on autonomic thermoregulation, enhancing the risk of hypothermia[30] (the original indication for chlorpromazine[31]). The manufacturers of clozapine recommend stopping 12h before surgery to minimise the additive sedative and hypotensive effects with drugs used during surgery. Otherwise, there are no significant concerns regarding continuing antipsychotics during the perioperative period, and there are more reasons to avoid discontinuation. There is an obvious risk of relapse of mental illness, but there is also evidence of an increased incidence of postoperative confusion[32] if chronic antipsychotic treatment is stopped.

CHAPTER 5

Recommendation: withhold clozapine for 12h before surgery. Restart when the next dose is due if blood pressure is normal. Other antipsychotics should be continued before, during, and after surgery.

MOOD STABILISERS

Asenapine inhibits CYP2D6 activity, so as described for some SSRIs and SNRIs, there is a theoretical loss of analgesic activity for some opioids. Carbamazepine is a potent CYP enzyme inducer (particularly of 3A4 and 3A5), so can reduce plasma concentrations of various anaesthetic drugs. Valproate may increase plasma concentrations of propofol, causing increased sedation and cardiorespiratory depression[17]. Valproate also reduces the glucuronidation of lorazepam[33], resulting in increased sedation[34]. Oxazepam and temazepam are also metabolised by glucuronide conjugation, but clinical evidence of an interaction with valproate is sparse. Lamotrigine presents no obvious problems.

Patients taking lithium are at risk of lithium toxicity postoperatively, principally due to blood loss (i.e. a reduction in circulating plasma volume), the initiation of NSAIDs for pain relief, and/or fluid shifts that result in fluctuating renal function. Changes in fluid intake or electrolyte fluctuations may also cause problems perioperatively. Many case reports describe postoperative lithium toxicity, particularly in patients undergoing bariatric surgery[35]. Preoperatively, patients may be asked to take liquid meal replacements to optimise pre-surgery weight loss and reduce liver size[35]. This alteration in dietary fluid and salt may affect lithium plasma concentrations. Postoperatively, lithium concentrations will be affected by changes in fluid intake. In vitro modelling of drug dissolution in Roux-en-Y gastric bypass[36] shows significantly greater dissolution of lithium compared with controls. Greater dissolution may contribute to the toxicity seen in clinical practice, and suggests a possible need for long-term reduction in lithium doses for patients undergoing this type of gastric surgery.

All patients taking lithium who are undergoing surgery should have plasma concentrations measured preoperatively to provide a baseline, and again postoperatively (within 24h). Patients having minor procedures that are not expected to significantly alter fluid balance, kidney function, or fluid intake can safely continue lithium. Some authors suggest that those undergoing major surgery, where there is the likelihood of large fluid shifts, blood loss, haemodynamic instability, and/or a high risk of perioperative acute kidney injury should discontinue lithium 72h before surgery[17]. This seems unnecessarily cautious and potentially risky for the patient's mental state. A more sensible approach would be to continue lithium up to 24h before surgery. Withhold lithium postoperatively, restarting only when kidney function is stable and lithium plasma concentrations are reducing (indicating that clearance of lithium has continued or resumed). For patients undergoing gastric surgery, plasma concentrations should be taken weekly for the first 6 weeks postoperatively, and then every 2 weeks for the remainder of the first 6 months. This is to allow adjustment of lithium dosing against changes in fluid intake that occur gradually in the months following gastric surgery. Monthly levels have been suggested for the remainder of the first year post-bariatric surgery, only after then returning to pre-surgery monitoring frequency[35].

Recommendation: carbamazepine, lamotrigine, and valproate can be continued perioperatively. Lithium should be stopped 24h before surgery and withheld in the immediate postsurgery period until renal function, fluid intake, and plasma concentrations indicate that it is safe to restart.

ANXIOLYTICS

There is an additive risk of CNS depression when benzodiazepines are given with anaesthetics or opioids, but the likelihood of withdrawal symptoms if chronic benzodiazepines are suddenly stopped is very high. Benzodiazepines should be continued during the perioperative period, including on the day of surgery[10]. Pregabalin and promethazine can be safety continued before, during, and after surgery.

Recommendation: continue anxiolytics perioperatively.

ADHD MEDICINES

The manufacturers of methylphenidate and dexamphetamine recommend withholding on the day of surgery if the use of halogenated anaesthetics is planned, owing to the risk of sudden blood pressure and heart rate increases. A blunted response to anaesthetic-induced hypotension is also reported, thought to be due to depletion of stored noradrenaline as a result of chronic stimulation of adrenergic and peripheral nerves[37]. However, clinical evidence suggests that stimulant drugs can be safely continued perioperatively[37,38] and routine monitoring for cardiovascular instability is sufficient. The amphetamines (dexamphetamine, lisdexamphetamine) are serotonergic so they increase the risk of serotonin syndrome if combined with serotonergic opioids. Morphine is preferable (see section on SSRIs and SNRIs).

Clonidine has analgesic[39], anxiolytic, anti-shivering, and anti-inflammatory properties. Some small studies have shown that initiating clonidine perioperatively can reduce the risk of myocardial ischaemia[40]. Larger studies have failed to confirm this, instead finding an increased risk of clinically significant hypotension and non-fatal cardiac arrest[40]. These findings may not be applicable to patients taking long-term clonidine (no studies have been done), since tolerance to the hypotensive and bradycardic effects develops over time. Abrupt discontinuation of clonidine causes rebound hypertension and tachycardia. Clonidine should be continued before, during, and after surgery[41].

There are no significant concerns with atomoxetine or guanfacine in the perioperative period.

Recommendation: withhold methylphenidate and dexamphetamine on the day of surgery. Other drugs can be continued.

CHAPTER 5

ANTIDEMENTIA MEDICINES

The cholinesterase inhibitors (rivastigmine, donepezil, galantamine) may prolong the effects of depolarising neuromuscular blocking drugs (e.g. suxamethonium)[42,43]. They may also reduce or reverse the effects of non-depolarising neuromuscular blocking drugs (e.g. pancuronium, rocuronium, vecuronium, atracurium, cisatracurium, mivacurium), requiring larger doses to achieve paralysis[42,44]. Withdrawing cholinesterase inhibitors risks worsening cognitive decline, so some guidelines suggest they can be continued during surgery if the likelihood of neuromuscular blocking agent administration is low[42]. Continuing cholinesterase inhibitors perioperatively does not appear to increase the risk of postoperative complications[45]. Current recommendations are to stop rivastigmine and galantamine 24h before surgery to avoid the interaction with neuromuscular blocking drugs. Donepezil has a long half-life (70h), so it takes 2–3 weeks to fully clear the body. Stopping treatment for this length of time is unlikely to be practical and may result in cognitive decline which is irreversible, even on restarting the drug[46].

Memantine is an NMDA antagonist, in common with ketamine. Concurrent use of these two drugs should be avoided. Otherwise, there are no concerns regarding memantine in the perioperative period.

Recommendation: donepezil and memantine should be continued. Rivastigmine and galantamine can be continued if neuromuscular blocking drugs will not be used during surgery; otherwise, withhold 24h before surgery and restart as soon as possible postoperatively.

SUMMARY

SSRIs and SNRIs	Continue
TCAs	Continue; avoid indirect-acting sympathomimetics
MAOIs	Discontinue tranylcypromine, isocarboxazid, and phenelzine 2 weeks before surgery OR continue but use MAOI-safe anaesthesia Stop moclobemide 24h before surgery OR continue but use MAOI-safe anaesthesia
Mirtazapine, bupropion, trazodone	Continue
Antipsychotics	Continue Withhold clozapine 12h before surgery. Restart when next dose is due if BP is normal
Mood stabilisers	Continue carbamazepine, lamotrigine and valproate Withhold lithium 24h pre-surgery and immediately postoperatively until renal function, fluid intake, and plasma concentrations are stable
Anxiolytics	Continue
ADHD medicines	Continue lisdexamphetamine, atomoxetine, and guanfacine Withhold methylphenidate and dexamphetamine on the day of surgery
Antidementia medicines	Continue donepezil and memantine Continue rivastigmine and galantamine if neuromuscular blocking drugs will not be used. Otherwise, withhold 24h pre-surgery

References

1. Roose, S. P. *et al.* Selective serotonin reuptake inhibitors and operative bleeding risk: A review of the literature. *J Clin Psychopharmacol* 2016; **36**: 704–709, doi:10.1097/jcp.0000000000000575.

2. Singh, I. *et al.* Influence of pre-operative use of serotonergic antidepressants (SADs) on the risk of bleeding in patients undergoing different surgical interventions: a meta-analysis. *Pharmacoepidemiol Drug Saf* 2015; 24: 237–245, doi:10.1002/pds.3632 (2015).

3. Gordon, N. C., *et al.* Interactions between fluoxetine and opiate analgesia for postoperative dental pain. *Pain* 1994; **58**: 85–88, doi:10.1016/0304-3959(94)90187-2.

4. Otton, S. V., *et al.* Inhibition by fluoxetine of cytochrome P450 2D6 activity. *Clin Pharmacol Ther* 1993; 53: 401–409, doi:10.1038/clpt.1993.43 (1993).

5. Kummer, O. *et al.* Effect of the inhibition of CYP3A4 or CYP2D6 on the pharmacokinetics and pharmacodynamics of oxycodone. *Eur J Clin Pharmacol* 2011; **67**: 63–71, doi:10.1007/s00228-010-0893-3.

6. Erjavec, M. K. *et al.* Morphine-fluoxetine interactions in healthy volunteers: analgesia and side effects. *J Clin Pharmacol* 2000; 40: 1286–1295.

7. Grönlund, J. *et al.* Effect of inhibition of cytochrome P450 enzymes 2D6 and 3A4 on the pharmacokinetics of intravenous oxycodone: a randomized, three-phase, crossover, placebo-controlled study. *Clin Drug Investig* 2011; **31**: 143–153, doi:10.2165/11539950-000000000-00000.

8. Grönlund, J. *et al.* Exposure to oral oxycodone is increased by concomitant inhibition of CYP2D6 and 3A4 pathways, but not by inhibition of CYP2D6 alone. *Br J Clin Pharmacol* 2010; 70: 78–87, doi:10.1111/j.1365-2125.2010.03653.x.

9. Lemberg, K. K. *et al.* Does co-administration of paroxetine change oxycodone analgesia: An interaction study in chronic pain patients. *Scand J Pain* 2010; **1**: 24–33, doi:10.1016/j.sjpain.2009.09.003.

10. Oprea, A. D. *et al.* Preoperative management of medications for psychiatric diseases: Society for perioperative assessment and quality improvement consensus statement. *Mayo Clin Proc* 2022; **97**: 397–416, doi:10.1016/j.mayocp.2021.11.011.

11. Hasnain, M., *et al.* Escitalopram and QTD prolongation. *J Psych Neurosci* 2013; 38.

12. Rochester, M. P., *et al.* Evaluating the risk of QTc prolongation associated with antidepressant use in older adults: a review of the evidence. *Ther Adv Drug Safety* 2018; 9.

13. Saraghi, M., *et al.* Anesthetic considerations for patients on antidepressant therapy – part I. *Anesthesia Progress* 2017; **64**: 253–261, doi:10.2344/anpr-64-04-14.

14. Bainum, T. B., *et al.* Effect of abrupt discontinuation of antidepressants in critically ill hospitalized adults. *Pharmacotherapy* 2017; **37**: 1231–1240, doi:10.1002/phar.1992.

15. La, M. K., *et al.* Impact of restarting home neuropsychiatric medications on sedation outcomes in medical intensive care unit patients. *J Crit Care* 2018; **43**: 102–107, doi:10.1016/j.jcrc.2017.07.046.

16. Li, M., *et al.* Impact of early home psychotropic medication reinitiation on surrogate measures of intensive care unit delirium. *Ment Health Clin* 2019; 9: 263–268, doi:10.9740/mhc.2019.07.263.

17. De Hert, S. *et al.* Pre-operative evaluation of adults undergoing elective noncardiac surgery: Updated guideline from the *European Society of Anaesthesiology. Eur J Anaesthesiology (EJA)* 2018; **35**: 407–465, doi:10.1097/eja.0000000000000817.

18. Sprague, D. H. *et al.* Enflurane seizures in patients taking amitriptyline. *Anesth Analg* 1982; 61: 67–68.

19. Kudoh, A., *et al.* Antidepressant treatment for chronic depressed patients should not be discontinued prior to anesthesia. *Can J Anesth* 2002; **49**: 132–136, doi:10.1007/BF03020484.

20. Stack, C. G., *et al.* Monoamine oxidase inhibitors and anaesthesia. A review. *Br J Anaesth* 1988; **60**: 222–227, doi:10.1093/bja/60.2.222.

21. Evans-Prosser, C. D. The use of pethidine and morphine in the presence of monoamine oxidase inhibitors. *Br J Anaesth* 1968; **40**: 279–282, doi:10.1093/bja/40.4.279.

22. Insler, S. R., *et al.* Cardiac surgery in a patient taking monoamine oxidase inhibitors: an adverse fentanyl reaction. *Anesth Analg* 1994; 78: 593–597, doi:10.1213/00000539-199403000-00030 (1994).

23. Noble, W. H. *et al.* MAO inhibitors and coronary artery surgery: a patient death. *Can J Anaesth* 1992; **39**: 1061–1066, doi:10.1007/bf03008376.

24. Taylor, D. M., *et al. The Maudsley® Prescribing Guidelines in Psychiatry*, 14 ed. (Wiley Blackwell, 2021).

25. van Haelst, I. M., *et al.* Antidepressive treatment with monoamine oxidase inhibitors and the occurrence of intraoperative hemodynamic events: a retrospective observational cohort study. *J Clin Psychiatry* 2012; **73**: 1103–1109, doi:10.4088/JCP.11m07607.

26. el-Ganzouri, A. R., *et al.* Monoamine oxidase inhibitors: should they be discontinued preoperatively? *Anesth Analg* 1985; **64**: 592–596.

27. Castanheira, L., *et al.* Guidelines for the management of chronic medication in the perioperative period: systematic review and formal consensus. *J Clin Pharm Ther* 2011; **36**: 446–467, doi:10.1111/j.1365-2710.2010.01202.x.

28. Jenkins, L. C. *et al.* Potential hazards of psychoactive drugs in association with anaesthesia. *Can Anaesth Soc J* 1965; **12**: 121–128, doi:10.1007/bf03004087.

29. Barry, B. J. Adverse effects of MAO inhibitors with narcotics reversed with naloxone. *Anaesth Intensive Care* 1979; 7: 194.

30. Kudoh, A., *et al.* Chronic treatment with antipsychotics enhances intraoperative core hypothermia. *Anesth Analg* 2004; **98**: 111–115, doi:10.1213/01.Ane.0000093313.16711.5.

31. López-Muñoz, F. *et al.* History of the discovery and clinical introduction of chlorpromazine. *Ann Clin Psychiatry* 2005; **17**: 113–135, doi:10.1080/1040123059100200.

32. Kudoh, A., *et al.* Effect of preoperative discontinuation of antipsychotics in schizophrenic patients on outcome during and after anaesthesia. *Eur J Anaesthesiol* 2004; **21**: 414–416, doi:10.1017/s026502150422511.

33. Samara, E. E., *et al*. Effect of valproate on the pharmacokinetics and pharmacodynamics of lorazepam. *J Clin Pharmacol* 1997; **37**: 442–450, doi:10.1002/j.1552-4604.1997.tb04322.x.

34. Lee, S. A., Lee, J. K. & Heo, K. Coma probably induced by lorazepam-valproate interaction. *Seizure* 2002; **11**: 124–125, doi:10.1053/seiz.2002.0590.

35. Bingham, K. S., *et al*. Perioperative lithium use in bariatric surgery: A case series and literature review. *Psychosomatics* 2016; **57**: 638–644, doi:10.1016/j.psym.2016.07.001.

36. Seaman, J. S., *et al*. Dissolution of common psychiatric medications in a Roux-en-Y gastric bypass model. *Psychosomatics* 2005; **46**: 250–253, doi:10.1176/appi.psy.46.3.250.

37. Fischer, S. P., *et al*. General anesthesia and chronic amphetamine use: should the drug be stopped preoperatively? *Anesth Analg* 2006; **103**: 203–206, table of contents, doi:10.1213/01.ane.0000221451.24482.11.

38. Cartabuke, R. S., *et al*. Hemodynamic profile and behavioral characteristics during induction of anesthesia in pediatric patients with attention deficit hyperactivity disorder. *Paediatr Anaesth* 2017; **27**: 417–424, doi:10.1111/pan.13112.

39. Blaudszun, G., *et al*. Effect of perioperative systemic α2 agonists on postoperative morphine consumption and pain intensity: Systematic review and meta-analysis of randomized controlled trials. *Anesthesiology* 2012; **116**: 1312–1322, doi:10.1097/ALN.0b013e31825681cb.

40. Devereaux, P. J. *et al*. Clonidine in patients undergoing noncardiac surgery. *New England Journal of Medicine* 2014; **370**: 1504–1513, doi:10.1056/NEJMoa1401106.

41. Mikhail, M. A., *et al*. Perioperative cardiovascular medication management in noncardiac surgery: Common questions. *Am Fam Physician* 2017; **95**: 645–650.

42. White, S. *et al*. Guidelines for the peri-operative care of people with dementia: Guidelines from the Association of Anaesthetists. *Anaesthesia* 2019; **74**: 357–372, doi:10.1111/anae.1453.

43. Crowe, S. *et al*. Suxamethonium and donepezil: a cause of prolonged paralysis. *Anesthesiology* 2003; **98**: 574–575, doi:10.1097/00000542-200302000-00040.

44. Bhardwaj, A., *et al*. Donepezil: A cause of inadequate muscle relaxation and delayed neuromuscular recovery. *J Anaesth, Clin Pharm* 2011; **27**: 247.

45. Seitz, D. P. *et al*. Effects of cholinesterase inhibitors on postoperative outcomes of older adults with dementia undergoing hip fracture surgery. *Am J Ger Psych* 2011; **19**: 803–813, doi:https://doi.org/10.1097/JGP.0b013e3181ff67a1.

46. Seltzer, B. Cholinesterase inhibitors in the clinical management of Alzheimer's disease: importance of early and persistent treatment. *J Int Med Research* 2006; **34**: 339–347, doi:10.1177/147323000603400401.

Chapter 6

Dialysis

CONTENTS

The Maudsley® Prescribing Guidelines for Mental Health Conditions in Physical Illness, First Edition.
Siobhan Gee and David M. Taylor.
© 2025 John Wiley & Sons Ltd. Published 2025 by John Wiley & Sons Ltd.

RENAL REPLACEMENT THERAPY

When a patient's kidneys fail, removal of waste products and excess fluid is performed by four main renal replacement therapies: haemodialysis, continuous ambulatory peritoneal dialysis (CAPD), continuous renal replacement therapy (usually performed in intensive care units), or kidney transplantation.

The most common type of dialysis is haemodialysis, where sessions on the dialysis machine are usually carried out three times a week for about four hours each. This is most often in hospital but can be performed at home. During haemodialysis, the patient's blood is removed from the body and then passed on one side of a semi-permeable membrane with dialysis fluid flowing on the other, before being returned to the patient's circulation. Small solutes can pass through the membrane; larger molecules cannot (e.g. blood cells, proteins). The process removes waste products and excess fluid in four ways:

- *Diffusion.* Solutes move from an area of high concentration to low concentration.
- *Ultrafiltration.* Fluid moves across the semi-permeable membrane under pressure.
- *Convection.* Solutes move with the fluid.
- *Osmosis.* Water moves from an area of high concentration to an area of low concentration.

Substances such as bicarbonate, often required in patients with kidney disease due to metabolic acidosis, can be added in higher concentrations to dialysis fluid, so they move the opposite way – across the membrane and into the blood. The aim is to replicate the filtering that happens when blood passes through the kidney glomerulus.

CAPD uses the peritoneum (which has a large surface area and is highly vascular) as the semi-permeable membrane. This requires a permanent catheter to be inserted to infuse the dialysis fluid into the peritoneal cavity. This fluid is drained off after a few hours. The process needs to be repeated a minimum of four times a day and is performed at home. An alternative is automated peritoneal dialysis (APD) where exchanges are performed automatically by a machine overnight.

This chapter deals with the use of medicines in haemodialysis, the process for which most data are available, but the principles may be extrapolated to other types of dialysis.

DEPRESSION

Prevalence

Depression is well known to occur in patients with chronic kidney disease, with prevalence rates possibly three times that of the general population[1]. Rates of depression in patients with kidney disease may exceed those seen in patients with other chronic illnesses[2]. When patients undergoing haemodialysis are screened for depression, rates are similarly high (one in four), with some studies finding that a large proportion of patients are undiagnosed and untreated[3]. The reason for this association is proposed to be tridimensional:

1 Inflammation associated with depression may contribute to the progression of kidney disease (it is possible that interleukin-6 plays a role in the pathophysiology of depression in dialysis patients[4]).
2 The burden of end-stage renal disease may lead to depression, and depression may increase the perceived burden of end-stage renal disease.
3 Depression may interfere with the patient's abilities to adhere to treatments and maintain good nutrition[5].

In common with other chronic physical illnesses, depression in end-stage renal disease may be associated with increased mortality[6-8], and the degree of risk may be linked to the severity of the depression[9].

Antidepressant choice

Despite the prevalence and impact of depression in patients undergoing dialysis, trials examining the efficacy and safety of antidepressants in this population are few. Where they have been carried out, they are mostly short (12 weeks). Many are non-randomised or open-label and are focussed on the use of SSRIs[10,11]. There are insufficient data to support the selection of any single drug over another in terms of efficacy in this population, so choice should be based on patient preference, extrapolation of data from non-dialysis populations, and safety. Given the significant burden of comorbidities often present alongside renal disease, the last of these is likely to be of key importance. It is worth noting that some symptoms commonly experienced by patients undergoing dialysis (fatigue, insomnia, poor appetite) may be caused by uraemia but overlap with diagnostic criteria for depression on frequently used rating scales in clinical trials[2]. This may also be pertinent when assessing response to antidepressant medication in practice.

Of particular note when choosing a drug for a patient undergoing dialysis is the possibility of contributing to the risk of an adverse cardiac event. Patients in end-stage renal disease are at an increased risk of cardiac side effects due to polypharmacy, electrolyte changes during dialysis, and the frequent presentation of cardiovascular disease comorbid with renal dysfunction. The riskiest time for cardiac events is the hours before, during, and after dialysis – fluid loading increases up to the time of dialysis, increasing the risk of bradycardia in the preceding 12 hours and increasing right ventricular pressure. This increases the risk of atrial fibrillation during dialysis. Further, if patients are taking rate-controlling medications for atrial fibrillation or hypertension that are removed by dialysis, then the risk of arrhythmia will be higher after dialysis[12].

The effect of antidepressants on QT is also important. A recent, well-designed, large retrospective cohort study examined more than 65,000 patients undergoing haemodialysis who were newly started on citalopram or escitalopram (designated as being QT-prolonging drugs by the authors) compared with patients starting non QT-prolonging SSRIs. It found a hazard ratio for sudden cardiac death of 1.18 for escitalopram and citalopram, with non-QT-prolonging SSRIs having no bearing on the risk of cardiac death[13]. Although the absolute risk is small (0.02% chance of sudden cardiac death in patients taking QT-prolonging antidepressants, compared with a 0.017% chance for those taking non-QT-prolonging drugs), this translates to one extra death for every 48 patients treated for a year. Subgroup analysis suggested an enhanced effect in the elderly, women, patients with pre-existing conduction disorders, and those taking other QT-prolonging medications. Neither class of antidepressant had any effect on non-cardiac death.

Overall, avoid citalopram and escitalopram in patients undergoing dialysis if possible, and especially if other risk factors for long-QT adverse outcomes coexist. TCAs should also be avoided due to their proarrhythmic effects (due to blockade of cardiac sodium and potassium channels), potential to cause bradycardia, and effects on cardiac contractility[14]. Mirtazapine or sertraline have been shown to be safe post-MI[15,16], a population at increased risk of arrhythmias, and would seem reasonable choices for patients undergoing dialysis. Neither are removed by the dialysis process (see below). Mirtazapine (and its metabolites) are predominantly eliminated in the urine, so severe renal impairment significantly reduces the overall clearance of the drug (by about 50%)[17]. Start at low doses and increase cautiously. Clearance of sertraline is not significantly affected by renal impairment and can be prescribed as in normal renal function[18].

PSYCHOSIS

For patients with schizophrenia, because of the chronic nature of the illness and the likely onset of psychosis (early in life) compared with need for dialysis (later in life), the question posed is perhaps more likely to be 'Can the pre-existing antipsychotic be continued?' rather than 'What antipsychotic can be newly started?' The answer to the first question must take into account the history of the patient response to antipsychotic medication, as well as their current response to antipsychotics.

Switching from an effective antipsychotic always carries a risk of relapse. This is a significant problem not only because of the obvious distress to the patient but also because the often chaotic nature of a psychotic relapse may affect the ability of the patient to comply with the dialysis regimen. Without dialysis, prognosis is inevitably dire, and so it may be worth pursuing psychiatric treatment strategies that may be less desirable in terms of physical adverse effects, in favour of stability in mental health.

It is also worth considering that manufacturers may advise against using their drugs in physical illness, including severe renal impairment, not because of direct data or biological theory about specific risk but rather because of a paucity of data in this comparatively small patient subgroup. This is not necessarily a reason to avoid use in clinical practice. Clozapine, for example, is contraindicated in severe renal impairment, despite renal clearance being barely relevant for its excretion. In fact, clozapine may be life-saving in patients with end-stage renal disease, as it is not a drug that can be replaced by any other antipsychotic – without it, relapse is almost certain. Maintaining treatment may allow dialysis to continue.

Depots

In principle, there is no direct contra-indication to using depots in patients who are undergoing dialysis. They may be preferable to oral medication for enhancing adherence, especially in a group of patients with a high physical-medication burden, and in whom maintaining psychiatric symptom stability may be essential to enabling physical health treatment. The main disadvantage of depots is that the drug cannot be quickly removed from the body if an adverse effect occurs or if the physical condition worsens.

There may be specific concern about the contribution of antipsychotics to QT prolongation risk during dialysis itself. For this reason, where possible it is preferable to use aripiprazole or paliperidone, as these drugs are shown to exert minimal effects on the QT interval.

In almost every case, depot doses for patients already established on treatment can be delayed by weeks, if not months, with little or no adverse consequence to psychiatric symptoms. If dialysis is expected to be temporary, and some return to physical good health is imminent, then it may be prudent to wait for this before giving the next dose. It is of course the case, though, that by the nature of the formulation design for 'typical' antipsychotic depots, active drug is not released immediately after a depot injection, but slowly and steadily throughout the weeks following the dose, so the strategy of delay may be more for the benefit of anxiety reduction in the clinical team rather than the patient. The enhanced risk of relapse for patients who do not receive their expected number of injections over the course of a year (e.g. where doses are repeatedly delayed or missed) should not be underestimated[19]. If doses are delayed, subsequent doses must be given at the originally scheduled time (check individual manufacturer's guidance for details).

THE EFFECT OF DIALYSIS ON PSYCHOTROPICS

The starting position for considering the effect of dialysis on the handling of drugs, including psychotropics, is to consider that dialysis does not restore renal function. Patients still have extremely poor to no kidney function in between dialysis sessions. Therefore, drugs that are not removed from the blood by the dialysis process should be used in terms of dosing and expectation of adverse effects, as they would be in someone with severe renal impairment. Even when drugs are removed by dialysis, this is not the same in practical terms as having working kidneys, as is evident when considering lithium (see below).

In principle, since drugs are not present in dialysis fluid, one would expect them to be removed by the dialysis process (remembering the principle of diffusion of solutes along the concentration gradient). Unfortunately it is not this simple, because removal also depends on molecular size, degree of protein binding, the volume of distribution, degree of water solubility, and plasma clearance. The combination of these factors make up the drug's 'dialysability'.

Dialysability

Several factors affect the likelihood that a drug will be removed by dialysis. Molecular size has an obvious effect, because the drug has to be small enough to pass through the pores of the semipermeable membrane in order to move from blood to dialysis fluid. Related to this, the proportion of drug that is bound to proteins is also relevant because protein-bound molecules are too big to pass through – only unbound drug can be removed. This also means that the proportion of drug that is available to be removed by dialysis may change if the patient's protein levels change. As a general rule, drugs that are more than 80% protein bound are less likely to be removed by dialysis than those with a lower proportion protein bound[20]. Drugs that have a high volume of distribution tend to have lower plasma protein binding (although this is not always the case), but are more lipid soluble. Therefore, they are distributed widely throughout tissues, and are present in relatively small amounts in the blood. This makes them less likely to be available for removal by dialysis (a volume of distribution of more than 0.7ml/kg is considered high in this context)[20].

Most psychoactive drugs are predominantly lipid soluble (they have to cross the blood–brain barrier for therapeutic effect), making them not only less available in the blood for dialysis, but also less likely to diffuse across the dialysis membrane where they are available. Dialysis fluid is aqueous, and so the more water soluble a drug is, the more likely it is to be pulled across the membrane for removal.

Finally, the overall metabolic clearance of a drug is a function of its renal and non-renal clearance. If the proportion of non-renal clearance for a drug is high compared with its renal clearance, then the impact of dialysis (which substitutes here for renal clearance) may not be significant, even if the drug is dialysed out. In this context, renal clearance of more than 30% is considered clinically important[20]. Only a few psychotropics reach this threshold.

Using these principles, the likely dialysability of a drug can be predicted. Broadly speaking, antipsychotics and antidepressants have high molecular weights, are highly protein bound, have high volumes of distribution and low water solubility, and are predominantly hepatically cleared. They are therefore unlikely to be removed during dialysis. This applies to the antipsychotics clozapine, olanzapine, aripiprazole, quetiapine, lurasidone, asenapine, cariprazine, haloperidol, chlorpromazine, zuclopenthixol, flupenthixol, and fluphenazine[18]. Antidepressants that are not dialysed are citalopram, escitalopram, sertraline, venlafaxine, duloxetine, vortioxetine, amitriptyline, agomelatine, fluoxetine, paroxetine, mirtazapine, nortriptyline, imipramine, lofepramine, mianserin, trazodone, and trimipramine[18]. The benzodiazepines diazepam, lorazepam, clonazepam, and midazolam are also not dialysed[18]. Carbamazepine is unaffected by dialysis[18]. For practical purposes this means that dialysis will not affect the clearance of these drugs, and dosing should be based on the patient having a creatinine clearance of <10ml/min.

It is not just the parent drug but also metabolites that must be considered. Hydroxylated and demethylated metabolites are renally cleared, as are glucuronides. These will accumulate if not removed by dialysis. Most metabolites are inactive, and therefore accumulation is of no clinical consequence, but some are not. Individual drugs that require particular consideration are discussed below.

Risperidone

Between 4% and 30% of risperidone is excreted unchanged in the urine (depending on an individual's CYP2D6 activity)[21], and it has a volume of distribution on the lower end of the antipsychotic scale (1–2L/kg)[18]. Some portion of it is dialysed, so one might assume that the dose available for clinical effect is actually lower than the dose given (as some will be removed by the dialysis machine), but the effect of this can probably be mitigated by giving the dose after, rather than before, dialysis. More importantly, the clearance of risperidone (and its active metabolite paliperidone) is reduced by 60% in severe renal impairment[18]. As a result, even though some proportion of drug will be removed on dialysis days, the recommendation is still to give lower doses (50% less) and increase at half the doses normally used, and more slowly[18].

Overall, the impact of a loss of a few milligrams of risperidone during dialysis (for patients taking 6mg daily, 1.5mg (25%) is removed during 5 hours of dialysis[18]) will differ for individual patients, but it seems unlikely to be of any significant consequence when considered over the course of a week (remembering that loss from dialysis is not a daily occurrence). Where published cases report plasma concentrations, they do not appear to differ significantly pre- and post-dialysis[22,23]. Nonetheless, dosing risperidone after dialysis and observing the patient for signs of relapse after dialysis days would be wise. If some instability in symptoms does appear to be related temporally to dialysis then it may be possible to 'top up' the lost drug with a small extra dose. The use of plasma concentrations to guide this may be helpful. Case reports describe successful use of risperidone depot in patients undergoing haemodialysis[22–24].

Paliperidone

Paliperidone is less protein bound than other antipsychotics (74%, compared with >90%), and is mostly excreted unchanged in the urine (59%)[18]. This may mean it would be a candidate for removal by dialysis, although other parameters might suggest otherwise (the volume of distribution, for example, is very high – 487L)[18]. Of note, clearance of paliperidone is drastically reduced in end-stage renal failure (by 71%) so if it were not removed by the dialysis process, extreme caution with dosing would be required. Scant data are available describing the use of paliperidone depot in patients undergoing haemodialysis, but where they are available (two case reports[25,26]) they show either no change in plasma concentration pre- and post-dialysis[26] or (in the absence of plasma concentrations) successful treatment of psychotic symptoms[25]. Overall, paliperidone appears safe to use in patients undergoing dialysis, but at reduced doses (reduce by at least half initially) to account for reduction in renal clearance, as it does not seem to be removed by the dialysis process.

Amisulpride

Amisulpride is much less protein bound than other antipsychotics (16%). About 50% is excreted unchanged in the urine, and it has a lower volume of distribution than many of the other antipsychotics (5.8L)[18]. It is poorly dialysed[18], so the effect of renal insufficiency

CHAPTER 6

is more problematic than the impact of dialysis itself. The clearance of amisulpride is reduced by a factor of 2.5–3 in renal impairment, with a corresponding 10-fold increase in the area under the curve in patients with moderate renal impairment[18]. The effect in severe impairment is probably even more marked, but few data exist, leading the manufacturers to recommend total avoidance. There are no data available describing use in dialysis. Extreme caution with dosing (start with minimal doses and/or extend dosing intervals) should be exercised if amisulpride is used in patients undergoing dialysis. Where possible, switching to a drug that is not renally cleared is preferable.

Sulpiride

Sulpiride is more protein bound than amisulpride (40%) but 90% is excreted unchanged by the kidneys (it is not metabolised)[18]. It has a lower volume of distribution than amisulpride (1.2–1.7/kg) and is partly dialysed[18]. Similarly to amisulpride, very cautious dosing should be used in patients with severe renal impairment (reduce by a third, and/or extend dosing intervals threefold). It is possible that some portion will be removed by the dialysis process, so give the dose after dialysis has finished. As with amisulpride, it is preferable to switch to a drug that is less likely to accumulate in renal failure.

Moclobemide

Moclobemide is 50% protein bound and has a volume of distribution of 1L/kg[18]. It is probably dialysed, but almost none is excreted in the urine. This means that dosing does not need to be altered for patients with renal impairment (since the kidneys are not involved in excretion of the drug), and dialysis should have no appreciable impact on plasma concentrations (this is confirmed by published data demonstrating no change in pharmacokinetics[27]).

Sodium valproate

Sodium valproate is metabolised extensively by the liver, and the metabolites are excreted by the kidneys. Valproate has a low volume of distribution (0.1–0.4L/kg)[18], but is highly protein bound (note the potential for increased free-fraction of drug if patients have low albumin levels). The high degree of protein binding makes it an unlikely candidate to be dialysed (except in overdose, where protein binding is saturated and a large amount of drug is freely available[28]), and some case reports show no changes in drug handling on dialysis days[29]. In contrast, other studies show that about 20% of the dose is removed by dialysis[18], depending on the dialysis efficiency (20% removal by low-efficiency dialysis, 42% by high-efficiency[30]).

Measuring plasma concentrations pre- and post-dialysis may be helpful in determining whether extra doses are required (a simpler solution would be to give the dose after dialysis). The presence of uraemia on non-dialysis days may increase the proportion of free drug for clinical effect[31], so it may also be necessary to check plasma concentrations between dialysis sessions, particularly if adverse effects appear. In reality, where valproate is used for psychiatric indications, there may be little clinical consequence to small transient changes in plasma concentrations[32,33].

Lamotrigine

Lamotrigine is primarily hepatically metabolised by glucuronidation, and the glucuronide metabolite is excreted via the kidneys. This metabolite is inactive, and so although excretion is impaired in renal failure, plasma concentrations of the clinically relevant parent drug are unaffected. Alterations in dosing for renal impairment should therefore be unnecessary, but the consequences of accumulation of the metabolite are unknown so the drug manufacturers advise caution in dosing.

There is disagreement in the literature about the dialysability of lamotrigine – some resources state that it is not removed by haemodialysis[18], but the volume of distribution is low (0.92–1.22 L/kg) and it is 55% protein bound[33]. A study of single doses of lamotrigine found 17% of the dose to be extracted by dialysis (although inter-patient variability was high)[34], and there is at least one published case of relapse of a previously stable bipolar disorder on starting dialysis, albeit without accompanying plasma concentrations[35]. The use of plasma concentrations to guide dosing is recommended, and giving the dose after dialysis (in preference to supplementing doses post-dialysis) is sensible[33].

Lithium

Lithium is an atom with low protein binding and a low volume of distribution. It is almost entirely renally cleared, has a narrow therapeutic index, and is predictably toxic at supra-therapeutic plasma concentrations. It is contraindicated by the manufacturers in severely impaired renal function. For some patients though, lithium is uniquely effective in the treatment of mania, depression, or suicidality, and so continuing it despite end-stage renal failure can be significantly beneficial. Doing so is not straightforward but is achievable. Several issues need to be considered, including when to give doses around dialysis times, how to manage the effects of any residual diuresis, and the rebounding of lithium concentrations post-dialysis.

After administration, lithium is distributed first into the extracellular fluid and to erythrocytes, and then to the intracellular fluid. An equilibrium between these two compartments is then reached after 5–10 days[36]. The process of dialysis removes 80% of lithium from the extracellular space[37], after which there is a gradual regaining of the equilibrium with the serum concentration as lithium moves from the intracellular stores to replace the extracellular dialysis loss. This takes 5–10 days, so if the aim is to achieve constant therapeutic plasma concentrations, some extra doses may be required during this period. The two-compartment model also explains the need to re-dialyse patients if dialysis is being used to remove lithium in overdose, as a second peak of lithium is observed after the initial peak is removed due to release of drug from intracellular stores.

Although dialysis is responsible for the removal of the majority of the lithium dose, there is also an influence of haematocrit. Dialysis cannot remove lithium from erythrocytes, and so the lower the haematocrit (packed cell volume), the higher the clearance of total lithium by dialysis, because a higher proportion is available in the extracellular space and therefore available to be dialysed[38].

The two final routes for removal of lithium are residual diuresis and sweat. Not all patients with end-stage renal disease are anuric, and where some diuresis still occurs, this will also lead to some lithium excretion. Lithium is also removed in sweat, so patients with hyperhidrosis may (at least theoretically) have lower lithium plasma concentrations[38].

The aim of dosing lithium in patients requiring dialysis is to achieve stable, therapeutic intra-dialysis plasma concentrations. There are several case reports describing a variety of methods for achieving this, and most do so by giving a single dose immediately after the dialysis only. This dose essentially stays in the body until the next dialysis session, where it is all but entirely removed, and another dose is needed. Where significant residual diuresis is present, authors have found plasma concentrations to be subtherapeutic using this technique – daily dosing may be required to take account of renal elimination[37]. What the initial dose should be can either be calculated using the volume of distribution, or a cautious initial dose can be given and maintenance doses adjusted according to plasma concentrations. Bjarnson and colleagues[39] describe the following method for calculation of a loading dose and then subsequent doses:

---

1 0.8L/kg * Bodyweight (kg) = Volume of distribution (Vd)
2 Vd (L) * Target lithium serum concentration (mmol/L) = Loading dose (mmol) given once after first dialysis
3 0.333 * Vd = Central compartment volume (CCV)
4 CCV * Target lithium serum concentration (mmol/L) = Maintenance dose (mmol) given after subsequent dialysis

---

Alternatively, other authors generally describe doses of around 400–600mg providing therapeutic plasma concentrations[40,41]. Patients who require long dialysis sessions (>5h) may require higher doses (more lithium is likely to be removed), and vice versa[38].

Plasma concentrations should certainly be used to guide dosing, but note that what constitutes a therapeutic level has not been defined for this population. A trough (predialysis) plasma concentration should be taken, and it is probably wise to aim initially for concentrations at the lower end of what is usually considered therapeutic, to account for the heightened sensitivity of patients with kidney disease to adverse effects, especially if uraemia is present (resulting in increased permeability of the blood–brain barrier). If signs of toxicity are evident, a post-dialysis plasma concentration may be useful (less lithium may be removed than expected). Time to steady state is difficult to predict because of the complications of fluctuating plasma concentrations around dialysis and the effect of plasma concentration rebound, but is probably at least a week[38].

Daily monitoring is required initially whilst maintenance dosing requirements are being established. Ensure the correct blood tube is used for sampling – some commonly used tubes for renal blood tests contain lithium heparin as an anticoagulant, which has led to spuriously high lithium plasma concentrations being reported[42]. Also worthy of note is that there may be an effect of the dialysate solution used on the amount of lithium removed during dialysis sessions, as well as the length of time the patient is dialysed for. Bicarbonate-based solutions may remove lithium from extra- and intra-cellular spaces more efficiently than acetate-based solutions[43], resulting in less effect of plasma concentration rebound and perhaps a lower post-dialysis lithium requirement.

In practical terms, a sensible approach would be to either calculate the loading and maintenance doses using the formulae given above or to start at a low dose (200–400mg) and increase cautiously. Whichever strategy is chosen, the dose should be given after dialysis only, omitting doses on non-dialysis days. Daily pre-dialysis lithium plasma concentrations should be taken for at least the first 2 weeks, or until the dose required to achieve stable therapeutic plasma concentrations is identified. Following this, the frequency can be reduced to dialysis days only. After stability is assured (three consecutive stable plasma concentrations)[41], monitoring can be extended to between one and three times monthly. Patients should be carefully observed for signs of toxicity or relapse.

Benzodiazepines

For benzodiazepines in general, the possibility for increased cerebral sensitivity in renal impairment and consequential excessive sedation and potential encephalopathy should be considered. Reduced protein binding in end-stage renal failure increases the unbound fraction of benzodiazepines, also increasing clinical effects (and adverse effects). For these reasons, smaller doses are advised for patients with kidney impairment. Dialysis itself does not affect the pharmacokinetics of the benzodiazepine parent drugs[44]. The glucuronide metabolite of lorazepam is removed by dialysis, but it is not pharmacologically active and therefore of no consequence. Clonazepam, diazepam, and midazolam, however, do have active metabolites, and in contrast to lorazepam, these are not removed by dialysis. There is therefore a risk of accumulation in chronic dosing. Single doses are unproblematic, but use lorazepam if regular administration is required.

SUMMARY

There is no psychiatric drug that is absolutely contra-indicated for patients who require dialysis. Even lithium can be managed safely and effectively with careful planning. If it is possible to avoid drugs that require adjustment in renal impairment (sulpiride, amisulpride, lithium), then this is preferable, but the priority must be to maintain stability of mental state in order to enable compliance with dialysis. If this requires use of drugs that are renally cleared and/or removed by dialysis, then patients should not be denied these treatment options.

Summary

Antipsychotics	Most antipsychotics are unaffected by dialysis.
	Prefer aripiprazole, lurasidone, or paliperidone due to minimal effects on QT interval.
	Cariprazine also has minimal cardiac effects, but note the long half-life of both parent drug (days) and active metabolites (weeks).
	Avoid amisulpride and sulpiride due to high proportion of renal clearance.
Antidepressants	Antidepressants are unaffected by dialysis.
	Avoid citalopram and escitalopram if possible due to small increased association with sudden cardiac death for patients on haemodialysis.

(Continued)

CHAPTER 6

Mood stabilisers	Carbamazepine is unaffected by dialysis.
	Small changes in plasma concentrations of sodium valproate and lamotrigine are possible; use plasma concentration monitoring and observation of symptoms to adjust dosing accordingly.
	Lithium is entirely renally cleared and removed by dialysis. If unavoidable, use is possible (see text for details).
Benzodiazepines	Prefer lorazepam. Other benzodiazepines have active metabolites that are not removed by dialysis and will accumulate.
	Use lower doses (expect increased cerebral sensitivity).

References

1. Palmer S. *et al.* Prevalence of depression in chronic kidney disease: systematic review and meta-analysis of observational studies. *Kidney Int* 2013; 84 (1):179–191. doi: 10.1038/ki.2013.77 [published Online First: 2013/03/15]

2. Shirazian S. *et al.*Depression in chronic kidney disease and end-stage renal disease: similarities and differences in diagnosis, epidemiology, and management. *Kidney Int Rep* 2017; 2 (1): 94–107. doi: 10.1016/j.ekir.2016.09.005 [published Online First: 2016/09/20]

3. Yeh C. Y. *et al.* Prescription of psychotropic drugs in patients with chronic renal failure on hemodialysis. *Ren Fail* 2014; 36(10):1545–1549. doi: 10.3109/0886022x.2014.949762 [published Online First: 2014/08/27]

4. Sonikian M. *et al.* Effects of interleukin-6 on depression risk in dialysis patients. *American Journal of Nephrology* 2010; 31(4): 303–308. doi: 10.1159/000285110

5. Katon W. J. Clinical and health services relationships between major depression, depressive symptoms, and general medical illness. *Biol Psychiatry* 2003; 54(3): 216–226. doi: 10.1016/s0006-3223(03)00273-7 [published Online First: 2003/08/02]

6. Farrokhi F. *et al.* Association between depression and mortality in patients receiving long-term dialysis: a systematic review and meta-analysis. *Am J Kidney Dis* 2014; 63(4): 623–635. doi: 10.1053/j.ajkd.2013.08.024 [published Online First: 2013/11/05]

7. Lopes A. A. *et al.* Depression as a predictor of mortality and hospitalization among hemodialysis patients in the United States and Europe. *Kidney Int* 2002; 62(1):199–207. doi: 10.1046/j.1523-1755.2002.00411.x [published Online First: 2002/06/26]

8. Wu P. H. *et al.* Depression amongst patients commencing maintenance dialysis is associated with increased risk of death and severe infections: A nationwide cohort study. *PLoS One* 2019; 14(6): e0218335. doi: 10.1371/journal.pone.0218335 [published Online First: 2019/06/14]

9. Saglimbene V. *et al.* Depression and all-cause and cardiovascular mortality in patients on haemodialysis: a multinational cohort study. *Nephrology Dialysis Transplantation* 2016; 32(2): 377–384. doi: 10.1093/ndt/gfw016

10. Natale, P. *et al.* Antidepressants for treating depression in adults with end-stage kidney disease treated with dialysis. *Cochrane Database Syst Rev* 2016; 5: Cd004541. doi: 10.1002/14651858.CD004541.pub3 [published Online First: 2016/05/24]

11. Nagler, E.V. *et al.* Antidepressants for depression in stage 3–5 chronic kidney disease: a systematic review of pharmacokinetics, efficacy and safety with recommendations by European Renal Best Practice (ERBP). *Nephrol Dial Transplant* 2012; 27(10): 3736–3745. doi: 10.1093/ndt/gfs295 [published Online First: 2012/08/04]

12. Weinhandl, E. D. Piecing together the risk of sudden cardiac death on dialysis. *Journal of the American Society of Nephrology* 2019; 30(4): 521–523. doi: 10.1681/asn.2019020185

13. Assimon M.M. *et al.* Comparative cardiac safety of selective serotonin reuptake inhibitors among individuals receiving maintenance hemodialysis. *J Am Soc Nephrol* 2019; 30(4): 611–623. doi: 10.1681/asn.2018101032 [published Online First: 2019/03/20]

14. De la Cruz, A. *et al.* Current updates regarding antidepressant prescribing in cardiovascular dysfunction. American College of Cardiology Jan 7, 2019, https://www.acc.org/latest-in-cardiology/articles/2019/01/04/07/59/current-updates-regarding-antidepressant-prescribing-in-cv-dysfunction.

15. Honig A. *et al.* Treatment of post-myocardial infarction depressive disorder: A randomized, placebo-controlled trial with mirtazapine. *Psychosomatic Medicine* 2007; 69(7): 606–613. doi: 10.1097/PSY.0b013e31814b260d

16. O'Connor C. M. *et al.* Safety and efficacy of sertraline for depression in patients with heart failure: Results of the SADHART-CHF (Sertraline against depression and heart disease in chronic heart failure) trial. *Journal of the American College of Cardiology* 2010; 56(9): 692–699. doi: 10.1016/j.jacc.2010.03.068

17. Timmer, C. J. *et al.* Clinical pharmacokinetics of mirtazapine. *Clinical Pharmacokinetics*, 2000; 461–474.

18. Ashley, C. *et al.* *The Renal Drug Database*. Boca Raton, FL: CRC Press; 2022.

19. Laing, E. *et al.* Relapse and frequency of injection of monthly paliperidone palmitate—A retrospective case–control study. *European Psychiatry* 2021; 64(1): e11. doi: 10.1192/j.eurpsy.2021.4 [published Online First: 2021/02/03]

20. Olyaei, A. J. *et al.* A quantitative approach to drug dosing in chronic kidney disease. *Blood Purification* 2011; 31(1–3): 138–145. doi: 10.1159/000321857

21. Mannens, G. *et al.* Absorption, metabolism, and excretion of risperidone in humans. *Drug Metabolism and Disposition* 1993; 21(6): 1134–1141.

22. Tourtellotte R. *et al.* Use of therapeutic drug monitoring of risperidone microspheres long-acting injection in hemodialysis: A case report. *Ment Health Clin* 2019; 9(6): 404–407. doi: 10.9740/mhc.2019.11.404

23. Batalla A. *et al.* Antipsychotic treatment in a patient with schizophrenia undergoing hemodialysis. *J Clin Psychopharmacol* 2010; 30(1).

24. Xiong, Y. *et al.* Injectable risperidone during hemodialysis. *Prim Care Companion CNS Disord* 2018; 20(2), doi: 10.4088/PCC.17l02212 [published Online First: 2018/04/28]

25. Lin, J-H. *et al.* Long-acting injectable paliperidone palmitate in a haemodialysis patient with schizophrenia. *Aus & NZ J Psychiatry* 2021; 55(8): 829–830. doi: 10.1177/0004867420952548

26. Samalin, L. *et al.* Interest of clozapine and paliperidone palmitate plasma concentrations to monitor treatment in schizophrenic patients on chronic hemodialysis. *Schizophrenia Research* 2015; 166(1): 351–352. doi: https://doi.org/10.1016/j.schres.2015.04.005

27. Stoeckel, K. *et al.* Absorption and disposition of moclobemide in patients with advanced age or reduced liver or kidney function. *Acta Psychiatr Scand Suppl* 1990; 360: 94–97. doi: 10.1111/j.1600-0447.1990.tb05346.x [published Online First: 1990/01/01]

28. Franssen, E. J. *et al.* Valproic acid toxicokinetics: serial hemodialysis and hemoperfusion. *Ther Drug Monit* 1999; 21(3): 289–292. doi: 10.1097/00007691-199906000-00005 [published Online First: 1999/06/12]

29. Kandrotas, R. J. *et al.* The effect of hemodialysis and hemoperfusion on serum valproic acid concentration. *Neurology* 1990; 40(9): 1456–1456. doi: 10.1212/wnl.40.9.1456

30. Araki, K. *et al.* Pharmacological monitoring of antiepileptic drugs in epilepsy patients on haemodialysis. *Epileptic Disord* 2020; 22(1): 90–102. doi: 10.1684/epd.2020.1139 [published Online First: 2020/02/08]

31. Dasgupta, A. *et al.* Diminished protein binding capacity of uremic sera for valproate following hemodialysis: role of free fatty acids and uremic compounds. *Am J Nephrology* 1996; 16(4): 327–333. doi: 10.1159/000169018

32. Baghdady, N. T. *et al.* Psychotropic drugs and renal failure: Translating the evidence for clinical practice. *Adv Ther* 2009; 26(4): 404–424. doi: 10.1007/s12325-009-0021-x

33. Bansal, A. D. *et al.* Use of antiepileptic drugs in patients with chronic kidney disease and end stage renal disease. *Sem Dialysis* 2015; 28(4): 404–412. doi: https://doi.org/10.1111/sdi.12385

34. Fillastre, J. P. *et al.* Pharmacokinetics of lamotrigine in patients with renal impairment: influence of haemodialysis. *Drugs Exp Clin Res* 1993; 19(1): 25–32. [published Online First: 1993/01/01]

35. Kaufman, K. R. Lamotrigine and hemodialysis in bipolar disorder: case analysis of dosing strategy with literature review. *Bipolar Disorders* 2010; 12(4): 446–449. doi: https://doi.org/10.1111/j.1399-5618.2010.00818.x

36. Chang, CWL, *et al.* Lithium use in a patient with bipolar disorder and end-stage kidney disease on hemodialysis: a case report. *Front Psychiatry* 2020; 11: 6. doi: 10.3389/fpsyt.2020.00006 [published Online First: 2020/03/03]

37. Engels, N, *et al.* Successful lithium treatment in a patient on hemodialysis. *Bipolar Disord* 2019; 21(3): 285–287. doi: 10.1111/bdi.12756 [published Online First: 2019/02/13]

38. Grüner, J. F. *et al.* Lithium treatment in maintenance dialysis. Review of the literature and report of a new case on hemodialysis. *Pharmacopsychiatry* 1991; 24(1): 13–16. doi: 10.1055/s-2007-1014426 [published Online First: 1991/01/01]

39. Bjarnason, N. H. *et al.* Optimizing lithium dosing in hemodialysis. *Ther Drug Monitor* 2006; 28(2): 262–266. doi: 10.1097/01.ftd.0000183386.35018.86

40. Knebel, R. J. *et al.* Lithium carbonate maintenance therapy in a hemodialysis patient with end-stage renal disease. *Am J Psychiatry* 2010; 167(11): 1409–1410. doi: 10.1176/appi.ajp.2010.10071009 [published Online First: 2010/11/03]

41. McGrane, I. R. *et al.* Lithium therapy in patients on dialysis: A systematic review. *Int J Psychiatry Med* 2022; 57(3): 187–201. doi: 10.1177/00912174211028544 [published Online First: 2021/06/29]

42. Topp S. *et al.* Lithium use in a patient on haemodialysis with bipolar affective disorder and lithium-induced nephropathy. *BMJ Case Reports* 2021; 14(7): e242841. doi: 10.1136/bcr-2021-242841

43. Szerlip, H. M. *et al.* Comparison between acetate and bicarbonate dialysis for the treatment of lithium intoxication. *Am J Nephrol* 1992; 12(1–2): 116–120. doi: 10.1159/000168430 [published Online First: 1992/01/01]

44. Ochs, H. R. *et al.* Diazepam kinetics in patients with renal insufficiency or hyperthyroidism. *British Journal of Clinical Pharmacology* 1981; 12(6): 829–832. doi: 10.1111/j.1365-2125.1981.tb01315.x

Chapter 7

Delirium

CONTENTS

The Maudsley® Prescribing Guidelines for Mental Health Conditions in Physical Illness, First Edition.
Siobhan Gee and David M. Taylor.
© 2025 John Wiley & Sons Ltd. Published 2025 by John Wiley & Sons Ltd.

INTRODUCTION

Delirium is a common neuropsychiatric condition that presents in medical and surgical settings. It is known by various names, including organic brain syndrome, intensive care psychosis, and acute confusional state[1].

Diagnostic criteria[2]

- There is a disturbance of *consciousness* (reduced clarity of awareness of the environment) with reduced ability to focus, sustain, or shift attention.
- There is a change in *cognition* (such as memory deficit, disorientation, language disturbance, or perceptual disturbance) not better explained by a pre-existing or evolving dementia.
- The disturbance develops over a *short period of time* (usually hours to days) and tends to fluctuate over the course of the day.
- There is often evidence from the history, physical examination or laboratory findings that the disturbance is due to concomitant medications, a medical condition, substance intoxication or substance withdrawal.

Tools for evaluation[3]

A brief cognitive assessment should be included in the examination of patients at risk of delirium. A standardised tool, the Confusion Assessment Method (CAM), is a brief, validated algorithm currently used to diagnose delirium. CAM relies on the presence of acute onset of symptoms, fluctuating course, inattention, and either disorganised thinking or an altered level of consciousness.

Clinical subtypes of delirium[4-6]

- **Hyperactive delirium**
  Characterised by increased motor activity with agitation, hallucinations, and inappropriate behaviour
- **Hypoactive delirium**
  Characterised by reduced motor activity and lethargy (has a poorer prognosis)
- **Mixed delirium**
  Features of both increased and reduced motor activity

CHAPTER 7

Prevalence

Delirium is present in 10% of hospitalised medical patients. A further 10–30% develop delirium after admission[4]. Postoperative delirium occurs in 15–53% of patients and in 70–87% of those in intensive care[7].

Risk factors

Delirium is almost invariably multifactorial, and it is often impossible to isolate a single precipitant as the cause[4]. The most important risk factors[4,5,8-10] have consistently emerged as:

- Prior cognitive impairment or dementia
- Older age (>65 years)
- Multiple comorbidities
- Previous history of delirium, stroke, neurological disease, falls, or gait disorder
- Psychoactive drug use
- Polypharmacy (>4 medications)
- Use of medicines with anticholinergic action

Discontinuation of chronic psychotropics, either intentionally or unintentionally, is not uncommon when patients are admitted for medical care. Failure to restart medication promptly (within days) increases the length of hospital stay[11] and incidence of delirium[12].

Outcome

Patients with delirium have an increased length of hospital stay, increased mortality, and increased risk of long-term institutional placement[1,5,13]. Hospital mortality rates of patients with delirium range from 6% to 18% and are twice that of matched controls[5]. In older people, the 1-year mortality rate associated with cases of delirium is 35–40%[7]. Up to 60% of individuals suffer persistent cognitive impairment following delirium, and these patients are also three times more likely to develop dementia[1,5].

MANAGEMENT

Preventing delirium is the most effective strategy for reducing its frequency and complications[7]. Delirium is a medical emergency; the identification and treatment of the underlying cause should be the first aim of management[14].

Non-pharmacological or environmental support strategies should be instituted wherever possible. These include co-ordinating nursing care, preventing sensory deprivation and disorientation, and maintaining competence[5,15]. Pharmacological treatment should be directed first at the underlying cause (if known) and then at the relief of specific symptoms of delirium.

CHAPTER 7

Common errors in the pharmacological management of delirium are to use antipsychotic medications in excessive doses, give antipsychotic medications too late, or overuse benzodiazepines[4].

General principles[4,5,16-19]

- Keep the use of sedatives and antipsychotics to a minimum.
- Use one drug at a time.
- Tailor doses according to age, body size, and degree of agitation.
- Titrate doses to effect.
- Use small doses regularly, rather than large doses less frequently.
- Review at least every 24 hours.
- Increase scheduled doses if regular "as needed" doses are required after the initial 24-hour period.
- Maintain at an effective dose and discontinue as soon as the clinical situation allows.
- Ensure that the diagnosis of delirium is documented both in the patients' hospital notes and in the patient's primary health record (include in discharge information).
- If it has not been possible to discontinue agents prior to discharge, ensure that a clear plan for early medication review and follow-up in the community is agreed.

CHOICE OF DRUG[20-23]

High-quality trials of pharmacological treatments for delirium are lacking. Available studies are often small, comprising heterogeneous populations and clinical outcomes, excluding patients with neurologic and psychiatric comorbidities[24]. Inevitably, they produce conflicting results. These problems mean that the results of meta-analyses must be approached with caution. For example, a network meta-analysis found a combination of haloperidol and lorazepam to be effective treatment for delirium, but this was based on a single study in cancer patients measuring effect on agitation, not delirium[25].

Antipsychotics

There is no high-quality evidence confirming that antipsychotics reduce the severity of symptoms in delirium or speed their resolution[26,27]. There is no good evidence to support the idea that antipsychotics shorten the duration of delirium, or improve quality of life. At most, antipsychotics may reduce some symptoms of delirium (e.g. agitation) in some patients[27]. Efficacy is by no means guaranteed[28,29]. More certain is the likelihood of adverse effects, particularly in patients who are elderly[30] or medically unwell. They are frequently unnecessarily continued at discharge[31,32]. For these reasons, it is vital that antipsychotics are used only to target specific symptoms, and stopped promptly if these symptoms do not improve.

Haloperidol[1,5,7,15,26,33-35]

In practice, haloperidol is the most frequently used drug for the management of symptoms in delirium[36,37] but it is important to note that superiority of haloperidol over any other drug has not been proven in clinical trials.

There are practical reasons for haloperidol to be preferred over other antipsychotics. It is readily available, cheap, can be delivered in a variety of ways (oral, intramuscular, intravenous, subcutaneous), and is available in a range of formulations (tablet, liquid, parenteral). It can be given in small doses, frequently, which may be preferable in medically frail patients at heightened risk of plasma-concentration related adverse effects. It is also a familiar drug to the non-specialist prescriber, a fact that probably increases both the likelihood of use and safety.

However, haloperidol may prolong the QT interval by blocking cardiac potassium channels[38], and as a result the Product Licence stipulates ECG monitoring. The specifics of the monitoring requirements are not consistent across different countries. In the UK, a baseline ECG is recommended when using haloperidol, regardless of the administration route. The US FDA does not require a baseline ECG, only recommending monitoring if haloperidol is given intravenously.

Haloperidol has been used in the management of delirium since at least 1978[39], and for many years the intravenous route was actually preferred over the intramuscular, specifically because it was thought to cause less cardiac stress[40]. Concerns about QT prolongation did not emerge until the early 1990s[41,42], when cases were reported in medically unwell patients that received intravenous haloperidol for delirium. Doses in these cases were high (50 to >1000mg/day). A warning from the FDA followed in 2007.

Since 2007, the majority of prospective studies have failed to demonstrate important QT prolongation with intravenous haloperidol[43]. Where QT prolongation does occur, it appears to only be at high doses[44] and to occur in patients with risk factors at baseline. A systematic review of reported cases conducted in 2010[45] found that almost all patients (97%) that experienced QT prolongation had other concurrent risk factors for Torsade de Pointes or QT prolongation, such as underlying heart conditions, electrolyte imbalances, older age, female sex or concurrent proarrhythmic drugs. Of these cases, 80% received cumulative doses of more than 10mg haloperidol. There were no documented cases of either Torsade de Pointes or QT prolongation at cumulative doses under 2mg. A large, multicentre, placebo-controlled RCT conducted in intensive care units in the United States found no evidence that either intravenous haloperidol or ziprasidone cause clinically significant QT interval changes or ventricular arrythmias in critically ill adults with delirium[46].

Similarly, studies conducted in medically unwell patients[47], including elderly populations[48], have shown that low doses of oral haloperidol (less than 2mg/day) do not result in QT prolongation. There may be a dose-related effect[49], but firm evidence for this is sparse[50]. Clinically significant QT prolongation is also uncommon with intramuscular administration, even at the higher doses usually used in schizophrenia[51].

It is not always possible to obtain an ECG in highly distressed patients. It has been suggested that if fewer than two risk factors for QT prolongation[50] are present, and doses are less than 5mg/day, then continuous cardiac monitoring for intravenous haloperidol is unnecesary[43]. The same guidance could sensibly be applied to other routes of administration. Withholding treatment or switching to a benzodiazepine in a patient with no significant risk of cardiac events purely for lack of a baseline ECG is probably not rational, particularly if the agitation poses significant risks[50]. It is also worth considering that switching to a different antipsychotic does not necessarily negate the risk of a cardiac event. Prescribers should be cognisant of the medicolegal consequences of prescribing outside the recommendations of the Product Licence/official labelling.

Olanzapine

The efficacy of olanzapine in management of symptoms in delirium has been demonstrated in several studies[22,52-56]. The sedative effects may be particularly beneficial in patients with agitated delirium[57].

Some experts have expressed concern about the anticholinergic effects of drugs such as olanzapine and quetiapine (both more anticholinergic than haloperidol, for example), reasoning that this may worsen delirium. It is possible that this explains the findings in some studies that olanzapine is less effective for delirium in older adults[55,58,59], although there are no trials that have been sufficiently powered to look specifically at this question.

The rapid-acting intramuscular preparation of olanzapine has not been formally assessed in the management of delirium. Intravenous[60,61] and subcutaneous[62] use of the intramuscular preparation has been described.

Quetiapine[22,63-70]

Along with olanzapine and risperidone, the effectiveness of quetiapine in improving delirium symptoms has been found in several network meta-analyses[27]. It may have a particular role in ICU settings[31,70,71], including in children[72,73], although findings are not consistently positive[74,75]. Note that QT prolongation is reported in some studies[50,76]. As for olanzapine, the sedative action of quetiapine may be useful in some cases.

Risperidone[22,54,55,77-84]

Risperidone is relatively well-studied in delirium[27], although not widely used in clinical practice, perhaps because it is less sedative than other atypical antipsychotics (e.g. olanzapine, quetiapine). A trial comparing risperidone with olanzapine showed that they were equally effective in reducing delirium symptoms but the response to risperidone was poorer in the older age group (>70 years)[55]. It is not apparent why this would be the case, other than age generally being a predictor of poor response to antipsychotics in delirium[59]. As discussed above for olanzapine, the differential effects of medicines in different age groups with delirium is understudied.

Aripiprazole[15,16,85-88]

Aripiprazole has a particular place in delirium management for patients with significant cardiac concerns, as it is less likely to cause QT prolongation than most other options[50].

Evidence of effectiveness in delirium, however, is extremely limited[89]. One small prospective study in elderly patients suggested that aripiprazole may be less effective than risperidone[88]. Agitation and akathisia may be a concern. It is undoubtedly less sedating that drugs such as olanzapine and quetiapine, and may have a role in hypoactive delirium for this reason[90]. Use of the rapid-acting intramuscular preparation has been described[91].

Other antipsychotics

There is very limited evidence for **amisulpride**[15,16,85,86], and its excretion via the kidneys makes monitoring of renal function imperative. **Lurasidone** is a theoretically useful option in patients at significant risk of cardiac events, as it has no effect on the QT interval[50]. To date, data are limited to a single open study in intensive care patients, which found it to be no different from quetiapine in efficacy or adverse events[92]. Lurasidone is very poorly absorbed orally unless given with a meal of at least 350 calories, which complicates its administration in delirious patients. There is some evidence for **blonanserin** patches[93-97], and transdermal administration may be particularly useful in palliative care or in patients who refuse oral treatments[98]. One small observational study found **perospirone** to be effective in patients with cancer, with fewer episodes of over-sedation compared with risperidone[84]. One pilot study[99] and follow-up RCT[100] of the use of intravenous **ziprasidone** in intensive care patients with delirium failed to demonstrate any benefit to duration of symptoms.

Summary

There is no firm evidence that any antipsychotic is either more or less effective than any other for any particular outcome measure in delirium. Adverse event rates are broadly similar for low-dose oral haloperidol, olanzapine, quetiapine, and risperidone[101]. There is no evidence to support switching between antipsychotics owing to non-response. Internationally, most clinicians opt for haloperidol first-line[36].

Benzodiazepines

Benzodiazepines increase the likelihood of developing delirium[102-105] and lengthen the time course of delirium[106], although the quality of evidence in this field is very low[107-109]. It is possible that the activation of GABA by benzodiazepines increases the release of deliriogenic neurotransmitters. Benzodiazepines also interfere with slow-wave sleep, which contributes to delirium[110]. One double-blind trial designed to compare haloperidol, chlorpromazine, and lorazepam in the management of delirium[111] found that patients who received lorazepam were oversedated, ataxic, disinhibited and confused. Ultimately lorazepam had to be removed from the treatment protocol. Benzodiazepines should be avoided if possible[108]. Do not abruptly stop long-standing prescriptions, as this is likely to precipitate withdrawal and may itself contribute to delirium[112].

In cases where antipsychotic treatment has been maximised but agitation remains and is interfering with medical care, benzodiazepines may be required despite the aforementioned negative effects. One randomised trial in palliative care[113] found that the

CHAPTER 7

addition of IV lorazepam (3mg) to IV haloperidol (2mg) led to an improvement in agitation compared with haloperidol alone, with no effect on length of stay or mortality. Although this trial did not include a lorazepam-only arm, it suggests a potential role for benzodiazepines for targeted symptoms (in this case, agitation), in combination with an antipsychotic. Longer-acting agents[102], continuous infusions[104] and higher doses[102,103] may confer more risk of developing or worsening delirium.

Other drugs

Cholinesterase inhibitors

Reduced cholinergic activity has been suggested as one of the possible causes of delirium[114], prompting interest in the use of cholinesterase inhibitors in treatment of symptoms. Studies using **donepezil**[115] have thus far been unconvincing. A study[116] which added **rivastigmine** to usual care (haloperidol) for patients with delirium in intensive care showed that rivastigmine did not decrease the duration of delirium. In fact, rivastigmine was associated with a more severe type of delirium, a longer stay in intensive care, and higher mortality compared with placebo. Use of cholinesterase inhibitors in the management of delirium is not recommended[117].

Alpha agonists

The alpha agonists (**dexmedetomidine, clonidine**[118]) sedate without impairing slow-wave sleep, which may explain their comparative superiority in some studies to antipsychotics for delirium outcomes[27]. Dexmedetomidine is only available in ICU settings because of the risk of cardiovascular adverse effects (hypotension), limiting use despite its efficacy in delirium being supported by two meta-analyses of RCTs[70,119]. Data supporting clonidine are less compelling[120,121] but some studies suggest superiority over antipsychotics in terms of time to delirium resolution[118]. Reported studies are almost exclusively in intensive care populations, although it can be given orally and any adverse haemodynamic effects (hypotension, bradycardia) can be managed by dose adjustments[122]. **Guanfacine**, an alpha agonist used to treat ADHD, has higher alpha-2 receptor selectivity than clonidine or dexmedetomidine. This makes it less likely to cause adverse cardiovascular effects[123]. To date, only one case series[124] and one retrospective chart review[123], both from the same group, describe use in delirium.

Valproate

Use of valproate in delirium has been described[125-130], usually in addition to other drugs and mostly in hyperactive or mixed delirium. The literature is limited to retrospective studies and case reports[131] and outcomes are not consistently positive. Hyperammonaemia and thrombocytopaenia are commonly reported. Few authors report plasma concentrations; where they are taken, most are below 50mg/L. Valproate is highly protein-bound, so the free-fraction may be elevated in patients with hypoalbuminaemia (not uncommon in medically unwell patients). This may result in a greater effect (beneficial or adverse) than expected at lower doses and total plasma concentrations. Dose and administration route (oral or intravenous) vary between published reports.

More data are needed before valproate can be recommended in place of other pharmacological options in the management of delirium, but it may have a place in treatment of agitation where use of other drugs has been exhausted. The dose should be titrated to symptoms, and loading doses can be used if rapid control of agitation is needed[132]. Do not increase the dose purely to achieve higher plasma concentrations, as this risks toxicity, particularly in physically unwell patients who are likely to have reduced plasma protein binding. It is essential to monitor for hepatotoxicity, pancreatitis, thrombocytopaenia, and hyperammonaemia[133].

Trazodone

Data supporting the sedating antidepressant trazodone as a treatment option in delirium are limited to retrospective chart reviews[134,135], secondary analysis of larger studies[136] or case series[137], all conducted in Japan. These reports suggest some potential benefits, possibly reflecting the importance of sleep on the development of delirium. Further studies are needed.

Others

One case report describes successful use of **phenobarbital** in hyperactive post-stroke delirium[138]. **ECT** has been employed in delirium, but published data are poor, almost entirely case reports, and mostly describe use in delirium secondary to substance withdrawal as a treatment of last resort[139].

Recommendation

There is insufficient evidence to strongly recommend any single drug treatment over others. Dexmedetomidine may be superior to other options[26,27,70], but use is limited to ICU settings. Treatment choice should be informed by the likelihood of interaction with coexisting medical conditions or other medications. In practice haloperidol is often chosen as a first-line agent, but other antipsychotics may be used. Benzodiazepines should be avoided. Valproate may be an option if all other avenues are exhausted.

PHARMACOLOGICAL PROPHYLAXIS[140-144]

Data relating to the use of medication to prevent delirium are sparse and conflicting. Most studies use low-dose haloperidol in patients deemed at high risk of developing delirium (elderly, post-surgery or ICU patients). Prophylactic low-dose haloperidol (around 3mg/day) was thought to reduce the severity and duration of delirium episodes and shorten the length of hospital stay in patients at high risk of developing the condition[145], but a more recent study in older subjects found no effect[34]. Higher doses

(>5mg/day) may reduce the incidence in surgical patients[146] but a large RCT found no benefit to mortality in critically ill patients[147].

Cochrane[140] suggests prophylactic olanzapine may be effective. One small RCT found some benefit to aripiprazole[148], another found none[149]. An RCT of quetiapine in older adults found no benefit[50], but another showed efficacy in surgical trauma patients in ICU[150]. A network meta-analysis suggested a possible effect for risperidone in cardiac surgery patients, but this was based on just two trials and a total of 227 patients[151]. One RCT found some benefit to prophylactic risperidone in elderly patients with hip fracture[152].

There is a growing body of evidence to support the use of the alpha-2 agonist dexmedetomidine in prevention of delirium for patients undergoing surgery[70,153], those who are critically ill[119], or those who suffered traumatic brain injury[154]. Studies that give doses perioperatively have shown a lower incidence of delirium compared with placebo[155,156] or other interventions such as ketamine[157] or melatonin[158]. This may be because of neuroprotective effects from the anti-inflammatory properties of dexmedetomidine, and/or improvement in pain control.

Rivastigmine may be effective[114,159] but Cochrane is dismissive[140]. Small, randomised trials have failed to find any benefit to donepezil[160-163], although a recent large retrospective study of critically ill patients with dementia[164] found those that were taking donepezil prior to admission had a reduced risk of mortality, shorted length of stay in intensive care, shorter duration of mechanical ventilation, and a reduction in delirium prevalence. Data are conflicting for melatonin[165-170], ramelteon[70,171-174], suvorexant[174-176], and combinations of these drugs[174,176] but they are at least well tolerated and may reduce sleep disturbance, which contributes to the risk of delirium[177]. A small study suggested a positive effect of minocycline (a drug shown to be neuroprotective in animal models)[178]. Avoiding benzodiazepine administration is probably helpful[179-181]. Some evidence exists to support non-drug measures to minimise the risk of delirium[182].

SUMMARY OF RECOMMENDATIONS

Drug	Starting dose	Comments
	In all cases, use the lowest possible dose for the shortest possible time	
Haloperidol[183,184]	Oral 0.25–0.5mg twice daily IM 0.25–0.5mg twice daily IV 0.25–0.5mg twice daily SC 0.25–0.5mg twice daily	First-line agent
Olanzapine[62,185]	Oral 2.5–5mg/day SC 5mg TDS IV 1.25–5mg twice daily	Useful option if sedation is required
Aripiprazole[186]	Oral 5–10mg/day	Use if significant cardiac risk. Less sedating than other options
Risperidone[187]	Oral 0.25–0.5mg twice daily	

Quetiapine[65]	Oral 12.5–50mg twice daily	Useful option if sedation is required
Lorazepam	Oral 0.25–1mg IM 0.25–1mg IV 0.25–1mg	Avoid use if possible Use only if antipsychotics are contraindicated and/or agitation is uncontrolled despite use of other agents
Sodium valproate[132]	Oral 125–250mg twice daily IV 125–250mg twice daily	Use if other agents have been exhausted Monitor for thrombocytopaenia, hepatotoxicity, pancreatitis and hyperammonaemia

References

1. van Zyl, L. Tc *et al*. Delirium concisely: condition is associated with increased morbidity, mortality, and length of hospitalization. *Geriatrics* 2006; **61**: 18–21.

2. American Psychiatric Association. *Diagnostic and Statistical Manual of Mental Disorders, Fifth Edition (DSM-5)*. American Psychiatric Association, 2013.

3. Inouye, S. K. *et al*. Clarifying confusion: the confusion assessment method. A new method for detection of delirium. *Ann Intern Med* 1990; **113**: 941–948.

4. Nayeem, K. *et al*. Delirium. *Clin Med* 2003; **3**: 412–415.

5. Potter, J. *et al*. The prevention, diagnosis and management of delirium in older people: concise guidelines. *Clin Med* 2006; **6**, 303–308.

6. Fong, T. G., *et al*. Delirium in elderly adults: diagnosis, prevention and treatment. *Nat Rev Neurol* 2009; **5**: 210–220.

7. Inouye, S. K. Delirium in older persons. *N Eng J Med* 2006; **354**: 1157–1165.

8. Saxena, S. *et al*. Delirium in the elderly: a clinical review. *Postgrad Med J* 2009; **85**: 405–413.

9. Naja, M., *et al*. Delirium in geriatric medicine is related to anticholinergic burden. *Eur Geriatr Med* 2013; 4 Suppl 1: S208.

10. Egberts, A., *et al*. U.S. Anticholinergic drug burden and delirium: A systematic review. *J Am Med Dir Assoc* 2020; S1525–8610(1520)30349–30342, doi:10.1016/j.jamda.2020.04.019.

11. Li, M., *et al* Impact of early home psychotropic medication reinitiation on surrogate measures of intensive care unit delirium. *Ment Health Clin* 2019; **9**: 263–268, doi:10.9740/mhc.2019.07.263.

12. La, M. K., *et al*. Impact of restarting home neuropsychiatric medications on sedation outcomes in medical intensive care unit patients. *J Crit Care* 2018; **43**: 102–107, doi:10.1016/j.jcrc.2017.07.046.

13. Miró, Ò. *et al*. Hyperactive delirium during emergency department stay: analysis of risk factors and association with short-term outcomes. *Intern Emer Med* 2023; doi:10.1007/s11739-023-03440-3.

14. Burns, A., *et al*. Delirium. *J Neurol Neurosurg Psychiatry* 2004; **75**: 362–367.

15. Schwartz, T. L. *et al*. The role of atypical antipsychotics in the treatment of delirium. *Psychosomatics* 2002; **43**: 171–174.

16. Seitz, D. P., *et al*. Antipsychotics in the treatment of delirium: a systematic review. *J Clin Psychiatry* 2007; **68**: 11–21.

17. National Institute for Health and Clinical Excellence. 2010. https://www.nice.org.uk/Guidance/CG103.

18. Donders, E., *et al*. Effect of haloperidol dosing frequencies on the duration and severity of delirium in elderly hip fracture patients. A prospective randomized trial. *Eur Geriatr Med* 2012; 3: Suppl 1, S118–S119.

19. Soiza, R. L. *et al*. The Scottish Intercollegiate Guidelines Network (SIGN) 157: Guidelines on risk reduction and management of delirium. *Medicina (Kaunas)* 2019; **55**: 491, doi:10.3390/medicina55080491.

20. Nikooie, R. *et al*. Antipsychotics for treating delirium in hospitalized adults: A systematic review. *Ann Intern Med* 2019; **171**: 485–495, doi:10.7326/m19-1860.

21. Li, Y. *et al*. Benzodiazepines for treatment of patients with delirium excluding those who are cared for in an intensive care unit. *Cochrane Database System Rev* 2020; **2**: Cd012670, doi:10.1002/14651858.CD012670.pub2.

22. Rivière, J., *et al*. Efficacy and tolerability of atypical antipsychotics in the treatment of delirium: a systematic review of the literature. *Psychosomatics* 2019; **60**: 18–26, doi:10.1016/j.psym.2018.05.011.

23. Devlin, J. W. *et al*. Clinical practice guidelines for the prevention and management of pain, agitation/sedation, delirium, immobility, and sleep disruption in adult patients in the ICU. *Crit Care Med* 2018; **46**: e825–e873, doi:10.1097/ccm.0000000000003299.

24. Martin, R. C., DiBlasio, C. A., Fowler, M. E., Zhang, Y. & Kennedy, R. E. Assessment of the generalizability of clinical trials of delirium interventions. *JAMA network open* 2020; **3**: e2015080, doi:10.1001/jamanetworkopen.2020.15080.

25. Wu, Y. C. *et al*. Association of delirium response and safety of pharmacological interventions for the management and prevention of delirium: A network meta-analysis. *JAMA Psychiatry* 2019; **76**: 526–535, doi:10.1001/jamapsychiatry.2018.4365.

26. Burry, L. *et al*. Antipsychotics for treatment of delirium in hospitalised non-ICU patients. *Cochrane Database Syst Rev* 2018; **6**: Cd005594, doi:10.1002/14651858.CD005594.pub3.

27. Sadlonova, M. *et al*. Pharmacologic treatment of delirium symptoms: A systematic review. *Gen Hosp Psychiatry* 2022; **79**: 60–75, doi:10.1016/j.genhosppsych.2022.10.010.

28. Andersen-Ranberg, N. C. *et al*. Haloperidol for the treatment of delirium in ICU patients. *N Engl J Med* 2022; **387**: 2425–2435, doi:10.1056/NEJMoa2211868.

29. Smit, L. *et al*. Efficacy of haloperidol to decrease the burden of delirium in adult critically ill patients: the EuRIDICE randomized clinical trial. *Crit Care* 2023; **27**: 413, doi:10.1186/s13054-023-04692-3.

30. Egberts, A., *et al*. U.S. Antipsychotics and lorazepam during delirium: are we harming older patients? A real-life data study. *Drugs Aging* 2021; **38**: 53–62, doi:10.1007/s40266-020-00813-7.

31. Boncyk, C. S. *et al*. Pharmacologic management of intensive care unit delirium: Clinical prescribing practices and outcomes in more than 8500 patient encounters. *Anesth Analg* 2021; **133**: 713–722, doi:10.1213/ane.0000000000005365.

32. Lambert, J. *et al*. Discharge from hospital with newly administered antipsychotics after intensive care unit delirium – Incidence and contributing factors. *J Crit Care* 2021; **61**: 162–167, doi:10.1016/j.jcrc.2020.10.030.

33. Fricchione, G. L. *et al*. Postoperative delirium. *Am J Psychiatry* 2008; **165**: 803–812.

34. Schrijver, E. *et al*. Haloperidol versus placebo for delirium prevention in acutely hospitalised older at risk patients: a multi-centre double-blind randomised controlled clinical trial. *Age Ageing* 2017; **47**: 48–55.

35. Zayed, Y. *et al*. Haloperidol for the management of delirium in adult intensive care unit patients: A systematic review and meta-analysis of randomized controlled trials. *Journal of Critical Care* 2019; **50**: 280–286, doi:10.1016/j.jcrc.2019.01.009.

36. Morandi, A. *et al*. Consensus and variations in opinions on delirium care: a survey of European delirium specialists. *International Psychogeriatrics* 2013; **25**: 2067–2075, doi:10.1017/s1041610213001415.

37. Matsuda, Y. *et al*. Current practice of pharmacological treatment for hyperactive delirium in terminally ill cancer patients: results of a nationwide survey of Japanese palliative care physicians and liaison psychiatrists. *Jpn J Clin Oncol* 2022; **52**: 905–910, doi:10.1093/jjco/hyac081.

38. Douglas, P. H. *et al*. Corrected QT interval prolongation associated with intravenous haloperidol in acute coronary syndromes. *Catheter Cardiovasc Interv* 2000; **50**: 352–355, doi:10.1002/1522-726x(200007)50:3<352::aid-ccd19>3.0.co;2-0.

39. Dudley, D. L., *et al*. Emergency use of intravenous haloperidol. *Gen Hos Psychiatry* 1979; **1**: 240–246, doi:https://doi.org/10.1016/0163-8343(79)90025-2.

40. Sos, J. *et al*. The intravenous use of haloperidol for acute delirium in intensive care settings. *Psychic and Neurological Dysfunctions after Open Heart Surgery* 1980; 196–199.

41. Hunt, N. *et al*. The association between intravenous haloperidol and Torsades de Pointes: Three cases and a literature review. *Psychosomatics* 1995; **36**: 541–549, doi:https://doi.org/10.1016/S0033-3182(95)71609-7.

42. Metzger, E. *et al*. Prolongation of the corrected QT and torsades de pointes cardiac arrhythmia associated with intravenous haloperidol in the medically ill. *J Clin Psychopharmacol* 1993; **13**: 128–132.

43. Beach, S. R., *et al*. Intravenous haloperidol: A systematic review of side effects and recommendations for clinical use. *Gen Hosp Psychiatry* 2020; **67**: 42–50, doi:https://doi.org/10.1016/j.genhosppsych.2020.08.008.

44. Sharma, N. D., *et al*. Torsades de pointes associated with intravenous haloperidol in critically ill patients. *Am J Cardiol* 1988; **81**: 238–240.

45. Meyer-Massetti, C., *et al*. The FDA extended warning for intravenous haloperidol and torsades de pointes: how should institutions respond? *J Hosp Med* 2010; **5**: E8–E16.

46. Stollings, J. L. *et al*. Antipsychotics and the QTc interval during delirium in the intensive care unit: a secondary analysis of a randomized clinical trial. *JAMA Netw Open* 2024; **7**: e2352034, doi:10.1001/jamanetworkopen.2023.52034.

47. Blom, M. T. *et al*. In-hospital haloperidol use and perioperative changes in QTc-duration. *J Nut Health Aging* 2015; **19**: 583–589, doi:10.1007/s12603-015-0465-4.

48. Schrijver, E. J. *et al*. Low dose oral haloperidol does not prolong QTc interval in older acutely hospitalised adults: a subanalysis of a randomised double-blind placebo-controlled study. *J Geriatr Cardiol* 2018; **15**: 401–407, doi:10.11909/j.issn.1671-5411.2018.06.003.

49. Miceli, J. J. *et al*. Effects of oral ziprasidone and oral haloperidol on QTc interval in patients with schizophrenia or schizoaffective disorder. *Pharmacotherapy: The J Hum Pharmacol Drug Therapy* 2010; **30**: 127–135, doi:https://doi.org/10.1592/phco.30.2.127.

50. Sadlonova, M. *et al*. Risk stratification of QTc prolongation in critically ill patients receiving antipsychotics for the management of delirium symptoms. *J Intensive Care Med* 2023; 8850666231222470, doi:10.1177/08850666231222470.

51. Harvey, A. T. *et al*. Intramuscular haloperidol or lorazepam and QT intervals in schizophrenia. *J Clin Pharmacol* 2004; **44**: 1173–1184, doi:10.1177/0091270004267807.

52. Skrobik, Y. K., Bergeron, N., Dumont, M. & Gottfried, S. B. Olanzapine vs haloperidol: treating delirium in a critical care setting. *Intensive Care Med* 2004; **30**: 444–449.

53. Sipahimalani, A. & Masand, P. S. Olanzapine in the treatment of delirium. *Psychosomatics* 1998; **39**: 422–430.

54. Duff, G. *Atypical Antipsychotics and Stroke*. Committee on Safety of Medicines, 2004. https://webarchive.nationalarchives.gov.uk/20141206131857/http://www.mhra.gov.uk/home/groups/pl-p/documents/websiteresources/con019488.pdf, 2004.

55. Kim, S. W. *et al*. Risperidone versus olanzapine for the treatment of delirium. *Hum Psychopharmacol* 2010; **25**: 298–302, doi:10.1002/hup.1117.

56. Grover, S., *et al*. Comparative efficacy study of haloperidol, olanzapine and risperidone in delirium. *J Psychosom Res* 2011; **71**: 277–281.

57. Kurisu, K. *et al*. Effectiveness of antipsychotics for managing agitated delirium in patients with advanced cancer: A secondary analysis of a multicenter prospective observational study in Japan (Phase-R). *Support Care Cancer* 2024; **32**: 147, doi:10.1007/s00520-024-08352-2.

58. Yoon, H. J. *et al*. Efficacy and safety of haloperidol versus atypical antipsychotic medications in the treatment of delirium. *BMC Psychiatry* 2013; **13**: 240.

59. Breitbart, W., Tremblay, A. & Gibson, C. An open trial of olanzapine for the treatment of delirium in hospitalized cancer patients. *Psychosomatics* 2002; **43**: 175–182, doi:10.1176/appi.psy.43.3.175.

60. Lorenzo, M. P., Burgess, J. & Darko, W. Intravenous olanzapine in a critically ill patient: an evolving route of administration. *Hosp Pharm* 2020; **55**: 108–111, doi:10.1177/0018578718823484.

61. Hassan, A. & Raschka, M. Avoiding a Poke: A case series of intravenous olanzapine in pediatric patients. *J Pediatr Pharmacol Ther* 2023; **28**: 752–756, doi:10.5863/1551-6776-28.8.752.

62. Elsayem, A. *et al.* Subcutaneous olanzapine for hyperactive or mixed delirium in patients with advanced cancer: a preliminary study. *J Pain Symptom Manage* 2010; **40**: 774–782, doi:10.1016/j.jpainsymman.2010.02.017.

63. Torres, R., Mittal, D. & Kennedy, R. Use of quetiapine in delirium: case reports. *Psychosomatics* 2001; **42**: 347–349.

64. Sasaki, Y. *et al.* A prospective, open-label, flexible-dose study of quetiapine in the treatment of delirium. *J Clin Psychiatry* 2003; **64**: 1316–1321.

65. Devlin, J. W. *et al.* Efficacy and safety of quetiapine in critically ill patients with delirium: a prospective, multicenter, randomized, double-blind, placebo-controlled pilot study. *Crit Care Med* 2010; **38**: 419–427.

66. Hawkins, S. B., Bucklin, M. & Muzyk, A. J. Quetiapine for the treatment of delirium. *J Hosp Med* 2013; **8**: 215–220.

67. Tahir, T. A. *et al.* A randomized controlled trial of quetiapine versus placebo in the treatment of delirium. *J Psychosom Res* 2010; **69**: 485–490.

68. Grover, S., *et al.* Comparative effectiveness of quetiapine and haloperidol in delirium: A single blind randomized controlled study. *World J Psychiatry* 2016; **6**: 365–371, doi:10.5498/wjp.v6.i3.365.

69. Mangan, K. C., *et al.* Evaluating the risk profile of quetiapine in treating delirium in the intensive care adult population: A retrospective review. *J Crit Care* 2018; **47**: 169–172, doi:10.1016/j.jcrc.2018.07.005.

70. Kim, M. S. *et al.* Comparative efficacy and acceptability of pharmacological interventions for the treatment and prevention of delirium: A systematic review and network meta-analysis. *J Psychiatr Res* 2020; **125**: 164–176, doi:10.1016/j.jpsychires.2020.03.012.

71. Williams, E. C., *et al.* Delirium in trauma ICUs: a review of incidence, risk factors, outcomes, and management. *Curr Opin Anaesthesiol* 2023; **36**: 137–146, doi:10.1097/aco.0000000000001233.

72. Caballero, A. *et al.* Quetiapine for the Treatment of Pediatric Delirium. *Ann Pharmacother* 2023; **57**: 1172–1177, doi:10.1177/10600280231154022.

73. Thielen, J. R. *et al.* Short-term effect of quetiapine used to treat delirium symptoms on opioid and benzodiazepine requirements in the pediatric cardiac intensive care unit. *Pediatr Cardiol* 2022; doi:10.1007/s00246-022-02980-3.

74. Cronin, M. T., Di Gennaro, J. L., Watson, R. S. & Dervan, L. A. Haloperidol and quetiapine for the treatment of ICU-associated delirium in a tertiary pediatric ICU: A propensity score-matched cohort study. *Paediatr Drugs* 2021; **23**: 159–169, doi:10.1007/s40272-021-00437-3.

75. Alghadeer, S., *et al.* Evaluation of the efficacy and safety of quetiapine in the treatment of delirium in adult ICU patients: A retrospective comparative study. *J Clin Med* 2024; **13**: doi:10.3390/jcm13030802.

76. Hanna, M. P. *et al.* Atypical antipsychotic safety in the CICU. *Am J Cardiol* 2022; **163**: 117–123, doi:10.1016/j.amjcard.2021.09.052.

77. Bourgeois, J. A. *et al.* Prolonged delirium managed with risperidone. *Psychosomatics* 2005; **46**: 90–91.

78. Gupta, N., *et al.* Effectiveness of risperidone in delirium. *Can. J. Psychiatry.* 2005; **50**: 75.

79. Liu, C. Y., *et al.* Efficacy of risperidone in treating the hyperactive symptoms of delirium. *Int Clin Psychopharmacol* 2004; **19**: 165–168.

80. Horikawa, N. *et al.* Treatment for delirium with risperidone: Results of a prospective open trial with 10 patients. *Gen Hosp Psychiatry* 2003; **25**: 289–292.

81. Han, C. S. & Kim, Y. K. A double-blind trial of risperidone and haloperidol for the treatment of delirium. *Psychosomatics* 2004; **45**: 297–301.

82. Hakim, S. M., Othman, A. I. & Naoum, D. O. Early treatment with risperidone for subsyndromal delirium after on-pump cardiac surgery in the elderly: A randomized trial. *Anesthesiology* 2012; **116**: 987–997.

83. Nguyen, P. V. & Vu, T. T. M. Efficacy and safety of risperidone in patients with delirium: The RIDDLE pilot study. *J Clin Psychopharmacol* 2024; **44**: 30–34, doi:10.1097/jcp.0000000000001770.

84. Inoue, S. *et al.* Safety and effectiveness of perospirone in comparison to risperidone for treatment of delirium in patients with advanced cancer: A multicenter prospective observational study in real-world psycho-oncology settings. *Acta Med Okayama* 2022; **76**: 195–202, doi:10.18926/amo/63414.

85. Boettger, S. & Breitbart, W. Atypical antipsychotics in the management of delirium: A review of the empirical literature. *Palliative & Supportive Care* 2005; **3**: 227–237.

86. Leentjens, A. F. *et al*, R. C. Delirium in elderly people: An update. *Current Opinion in Psychiatry* 2005; **18**: 325–330.

87. Boettger, S., *et al.* Aripiprazole and haloperidol in the treatment of delirium. *Aust NZ J Psychiatry* 2011; **45**: 477–482.

88. Sugawara, H. *et al.* Prospective clinical intervention study of aripiprazole and risperidone in the management of postoperative delirium in elderly patients after cardiovascular surgery. *Psychiatry Clin Neurosci* 2022; **76**: 531–533, doi:10.1111/pcn.13446.

89. Jarosz, M. *et al.* Efficacy and safety of aripiprazole in the treatment of delirium. *Psychiatria Polska* 2023; 1–10, doi:10.12740/PP/OnlineFirst/156262.

90. Lodewijckx, E., *et al.* Pharmacologic treatment for hypoactive delirium in adult patients: A brief report of the literature. *J Am Med Dir Assoc* 2021; **22**: 1313–1316.e1312, doi:10.1016/j.jamda.2020.12.037.

91. Martinotti, G. *et al.* Psychomotor agitation and hyperactive delirium in COVID-19 patients treated with aripiprazole 9.75mg/1.3ml immediate release. *Psychopharmacology (Berlin)* 2020; 1–5, doi:10.1007/s00213-020-05644-3.

92. Fox, M. A., *et al.* Comparison of lurasidone versus quetiapine for the treatment of delirium in critically ill patients. *J Intensive Care Med* 2020; **35**: 394–399, doi:10.1177/0885066617754187.

93. Nishiofuku, H. *et al.* Successful Management of Terminal Delirium With Transdermal Blonanserin Patch in a Terminally Ill Cancer Patient. *J Palliat Med* 2024; doi:10.1089/jpm.2023.0584.

94. Ando, K., *et al.* Efficacy of blonanserin transdermal patch on terminal delirium in patients with respiratory diseases. *Respir Investig* 2023; 61: 240–246, doi:10.1016/j.resinv.2023.01.006.

95. Andoh, H. *et al.* Case of delirium complicated with pneumonia that improved with blonanserin administration. *Psychiatry Clin Neurosci* 2010; 64: 588–589, doi:10.1111/j.1440-1819.2010.02124.x.

96. Kato, K. *et al.* Blonanserin for the treatment of delirium patients at an emergency medical care center: an open-label study. *Asian J Psychiatr* 2013; 6: 182–183, doi:10.1016/j.ajp.2012.09.003.

97. Kato, K. *et al.* Blonanserin in the treatment of delirium. *Psychiatry Clin Neurosci* 2011; 65: 389–391, doi:10.1111/j.1440-1819.2011.02213.x.

98. Hatta, K., Usui, C. & Nakamura, H. Acceptability of transdermal antipsychotic patches by patients who refuse oral medication and their effectiveness in preventing recurrence of delirium: a retrospective observational study. *Int Clin Psychopharmacol* 2023; 38: 23–27, doi:10.1097/yic.0000000000000428.

99. Girard, T. D. *et al.* Feasibility, efficacy, and safety of antipsychotics for intensive care unit delirium: The MIND randomized, placebo-controlled trial. *Crit Care Med* 2010; 38(2): 428–437, doi:10.1097/CCM.0b013e3181c58715.

100. Girard, T. D. *et al.* Haloperidol and Ziprasidone for Treatment of Delirium in Critical Illness. *N Engl J Med* 2018; 379: 2506–2516, doi:10.1056/NEJMoa1808217.

101. Kim, D. H. *et al.* Comparative safety analysis of oral antipsychotics for in-hospital adverse clinical events in older adults after major surgery: a nationwide cohort study. *Annals of Internal Medicine* 2023; 176: 1153–1162, doi:10.7326/m22-3021.

102. Marcantonio, E. R. *et al.* The relationship of postoperative delirium with psychoactive medications. *JAMA* 1994; 272: 1518–1522.

103. Pandharipande, P. *et al.* Lorazepam is an independent risk factor for transitioning to delirium in intensive care unit patients. *Anesthesiology* 2006; 104: 21–26, doi:10.1097/00000542-200601000-00005.

104. Zaal, I. J. *et al.* Benzodiazepine-associated delirium in critically ill adults. *Intensive Care Med* 2015; 41: 2130–2137, doi:10.1007/s00134-015-4063-z.

105. He, M. *et al.* Risk Factors for Postanesthetic Emergence Delirium in Adults: A Systematic Review and Meta-analysis. *J Neurosurg Anesthesiol*, 2023; doi:10.1097/ana.0000000000000942.

106. Wang, H. *et al.* Sedative drugs used for mechanically ventilated patients in intensive care units: a systematic review and network meta-analysis. *Curr Med Res Opin* 2019; 35: 435–446, doi:10.1080/03007995.2018.1509573.

107. Wang, E. *et al.* Effect of perioperative benzodiazepine use on intraoperative awareness and postoperative delirium: a systematic review and meta-analysis of randomised controlled trials and observational studies. *Br J Anaesth* 2023 Aug; 131(2): 302–313.

108. Lonergan, E., *et al.* Benzodiazepines for delirium. *Cochrane Database Syst Rev* 2009: Cd006379, doi:10.1002/14651858.CD006379.pub3.

109. Reisinger, M., *et al.* Delirium-associated medication in people at risk: A systematic update review, meta-analyses, and GRADE-profiles. *Acta Psychiatr Scand* 2023; 147: 16–42, doi:10.1111/acps.13505.

110. van der Hoeven, A. E. *et al.* Sleep in the intensive and intermediate care units: Exploring related factors of delirium, benzodiazepine use and mortality. *Intensive Critical Care Nursing* 2024; 81: 103603, doi:10.1016/j.iccn.2023.103603.

111. Breitbart, W. *et al.* A double-blind trial of haloperidol, chlorpromazine, and lorazepam in the treatment of delirium in hospitalized AIDS patients. *Focus* 2025; 153: 231–340.

112. Omichi, C. *et al.* Association between discontinuation of benzodiazepine receptor agonists and post-operative delirium among inpatients with liaison intervention: A retrospective cohort study. *Compr Psychiatry* 2021; 104: 152216, doi:10.1016/j.comppsych.2020.152216.

113. Hui, D. *et al.* Effect of lorazepam with haloperidol vs haloperidol alone on agitated delirium in patients with advanced cancer receiving palliative care: A randomized clinical trial. *JAMA* 2017; 318: 1047–1056, doi:10.1001/jama.2017.11468.

114. Massoudi, N. *et al.* The impact of rivastigmine on post-surgical delirium and cognitive impairment: A randomized clinical trial. *Int J Geriatr Psychiatry* 2023; 38: e5970, doi:10.1002/gps.5970.

115. Sampson, E. L. *et al.* A randomized, double-blind, placebo-controlled trial of donepezil hydrochloride (Aricept) for reducing the incidence of postoperative delirium after elective total hip replacement. *Int J Geriatr Psychiatry* 2007; 22: 343–349.

116. van Eijk, M. M. *et al.* Effect of rivastigmine as an adjunct to usual care with haloperidol on duration of delirium and mortality in critically ill patients: a multicentre, double-blind, placebo-controlled randomised trial. *Lancet* 2010; 376: 1829–1837.

117. Yu, A. *et al.* Cholinesterase inhibitors for the treatment of delirium in non-ICU settings. *Cochrane Database Syst Rev* 2018; 6: Cd012494, doi:10.1002/14651858.CD012494.pub2.

118. Wu, T. T., *et al.* Research letter: Clonidine is associated with faster first resolution of incident ICU delirium than antipsychotics. *Journal of Critical Care* 2024; 79: 154433, doi:https://doi.org/10.1016/j.jcrc.2023.154433.

119. Burry, L. D. *et al.* Pharmacological and non-pharmacological interventions to prevent delirium in critically ill patients: a systematic review and network meta-analysis. *Intensive Care Medicine* 2021; 47: 943–960, doi:10.1007/s00134-021-06490-3.

120. Smit, L., Dijkstra-Kersten, S. M. A., Zaal, I. J., van der Jagt, M. & Slooter, A. J. C. Haloperidol, clonidine and resolution of delirium in critically ill patients: a prospective cohort study. *Intensive Care Med* 2021; 47: 316–324, doi:10.1007/s00134-021-06355-9.

121. Hov, K. R. *et al.* The Oslo Study of Clonidine in Elderly Patients with Delirium; LUCID: a randomised placebo-controlled trial. *Int J Geriatr Psychiatry* 2019; 34: 974–981, doi:https://doi.org/10.1002/gps.5098.

122. Hov, K. R. *et al.* The use of clonidine in elderly patients with delirium; pharmacokinetics and hemodynamic responses. *BMC Pharmacol Toxicol* 2018; 19: 29, doi:10.1186/s40360-018-0218-1.

123. Jiang, S. *et al*. A retrospective analysis of guanfacine for the pharmacological management of delirium. *Cureus* 2023; **15**: e33393, doi:10.7759/cureus.33393.

124. Jiang, S., *et al*. Guanfacine for hyperactive delirium: A case series. *J Acad Consult Liaison Psychiatry* 2021; **62**: 83–88, doi:10.1016/j.psym.2020.10.003.

125. Sher, Y., *et al*. Adjunctive valproic acid in management-refractory hyperactive delirium: A case series and rationale. *J Neuropsychiatry Clin Neurosci* 2015; **27**: 365–370, doi:10.1176/appi.neuropsych.14080190.

126. Gagnon, D. J. *et al*. Valproate for agitation in critically ill patients: A retrospective study. *J Crit Care* 2017; **37**: 119–125, doi:10.1016/j.jcrc.2016.09.006.

127. Crowley, K. E., *et al*. Valproic acid for the management of agitation and delirium in the intensive care setting: A retrospective analysis. *Clin Ther* 2020; **42**: e65–e73, doi:10.1016/j.clinthera.2020.02.007.

128. Quinn, N. J., *et al*. Prescribing practices of valproic acid for agitation and delirium in the intensive care unit. *Ann. Pharmacother* 2020; 1060028020947173, doi:10.1177/1060028020947173.

129. Quinn, N. J., *et al*. Prescribing practices of valproic acid for agitation and delirium in the intensive care unit. *Ann Pharmacother* 2021; **55**: 311–317, doi:10.1177/1060028020947173.

130. Swayngim, R., *et al*. Use of valproic acid for the management of delirium and agitation in the intensive care unit. *J Pharm Pract* 2024; **37**: 118–122, doi:10.1177/08971900221128636.

131. Cuartas, C. F., *et al*. Valproic acid in the management of delirium. *Am J Hosp Palliat Care* 2022; **39**: 562–569, doi:10.1177/10499091211038371.

132. Sher, Y., *et al*. Valproic acid for treatment of hyperactive or mixed delirium: Rationale and literature review. *Psychosomatics* 2015; **56**: 615–625, doi:10.1016/j.psym.2015.09.008.

133. Gagnon, D. J., *et al*. Repurposing valproate, enteral clonidine, and phenobarbital for comfort in adult ICU patients: a literature review with practical considerations. *Pharmacotherapy* 2017; **37**: 1309–1321, doi:10.1002/phar.2017.

134. Kawano, S. *et al*. Trazodone and mianserin for delirium: A retrospective chart review. *J Clin Psychopharmacol* 2022; **42**: 560–564, doi:10.1097/jcp.0000000000001619.

135. Wada, K., *et al*. First- and second-line pharmacological treatment for delirium in general hospital setting – Retrospective analysis. *Asian J Psychiatr* 2018; **32**: 50–53, doi:10.1016/j.ajp.2017.11.028.

136. Maeda, I. *et al*. Low-dose trazodone for delirium in patients with cancer who received specialist palliative care: A multicenter prospective study. *J Palliat Med* 2021; **24**: 914–918, doi:10.1089/jpm.2020.0610.

137. Okamoto, Y. *et al*. Trazodone in the treatment of delirium. *J Clin Psychopharmacol* 1999; **19**: 280–282, doi:10.1097/00004714-199906000-00018.

138. Hilbert, M. T., Henkel, N. D., Spetz, S. L. & Malaiyandi, D. P. The Rising Status of Phenobarbital: A Case for Use in Severe Refractory Hyperactive Poststroke Delirium. *Neurologist* 2023; **28**: 123–125, doi:10.1097/nrl.0000000000000441.

139. Lupke, K. *et al*. A systematic review of modified electroconvulsive therapy (ECT) to treat delirium. *Acta Psychiatrica Scandinavica* 2023; **147**: 403–419, doi:https://doi.org/10.1111/acps.13492.

140. Siddiqi, N. *et al*. Interventions for preventing delirium in hospitalised non-ICU patients. *Cochrane Database System Rev* 2016; **3**: Cd005563, doi:10.1002/14651858.CD005563.pub3.

141. Santos, E. *et al*. Effectiveness of haloperidol prophylaxis in critically ill patients with a high risk of delirium: A systematic review. *JBI Database of Systematic Reviews and Implementation Reports* 2017; **15**: 1440–1472, doi:10.11124/jbisrir-2017-003391.

142. Fok, M. C. *et al*. Do antipsychotics prevent postoperative delirium? A systematic review and meta-analysis. *Int. J Geriatr Psychiatry* 2015; **30**: 333–344, doi:10.1002/gps.4240.

143. Schrijver, E. J., *et al*. Efficacy and safety of haloperidol for in-hospital delirium prevention and treatment: A systematic review of current evidence. *Eur. J. Intern. Med.* 2016; **27**: 14–23, doi:10.1016/j.ejim.2015.10.012.

144. Oh, E. S. *et al*. Antipsychotics for preventing delirium in hospitalized adults: A systematic review. *Ann Intern Med* 2019; **171**: 474–484, doi:10.7326/m19-1859.

145. van den Boogaard, M., *et al*. Haloperidol prophylaxis in critically ill patients with a high risk for delirium. *Crit Care* 2013; **17**: R9, doi:10.1186/cc11933.

146. Shen, Y. Z., *et al*. Effects of haloperidol on delirium in adult patients: A systematic review and meta-analysis. *Med. Princ. Pract.* 2018; **27**: 250–259, doi:10.1159/000488243.

147. van den Boogaard, M. *et al*. Effect of haloperidol on survival among critically ill adults with a high risk of delirium: The REDUCE randomized clinical trial. *JAMA* 2018; **319**: 680–690, doi:10.1001/jama.2018.0160.

148. Mokhtari, M. *et al*. Aripiprazole for prevention of delirium in the neurosurgical intensive care unit: a double-blind, randomized, placebo-controlled study. *Eur J Clin Pharmacol* 2020; **76**: 491–499, doi:10.1007/s00228-019-02802-1.

149. Nouri, M., *et al*. Evaluation of the effect of aripiprazole supplementation in the prevention of delirium in patients admitted to the general intensive care unit. *Adv Biomed Res* 2023; **12**: 198, doi:10.4103/abr.abr_314_21.

150. Abraham, M. P. *et al*. Quetiapine for delirium prophylaxis in high-risk critically ill patients. *Surgeon* 2021; **19**: 65–71, doi:10.1016/j.surge.2020.02.002.

151. Meco, M., *et al*. Pharmacological prevention of postoperative delirium in patients undergoing cardiac surgery: a bayesian network meta-analysis. *J Anesth* 2023; **37**: 294–310, doi:10.1007/s00540-023-03170-y.

152. Jing, G. W. *et al*. Early intervention of perioperative delirium in older patients (>60 years) with hip fracture: A randomized controlled study. *Orthop Surg* 2022; **14**: 885–891, doi:10.1111/os.13244.

CHAPTER 7

153. Lin, C., *et al.* Effect of dexmedetomidine on delirium in elderly surgical patients: A meta-analysis of randomized controlled trials. *Ann Pharmacother* 2021; **55**: 624–636, doi:10.1177/1060028020951954.

154. Huang, Y. Q. *et al.* Prevention and treatment of traumatic brain injury-related delirium: a systematic review. *J Neurol* 2023; **270**: 5966–5987, doi:10.1007/s00415-023-11889-7.

155. Likhvantsev, V. V. *et al.* Perioperative dexmedetomidine supplement decreases delirium incidence after adult cardiac surgery: A randomized, double-blind, controlled study. *J Cardiothorac Vasc Anesth* 2021; **35**: 449–457, doi:10.1053/j.jvca.2020.02.035.

156. He, H. *et al.* The effect of intranasal dexmedetomidine on emergence delirium prevention in pediatric ambulatory dental rehabilitation under general anesthesia: A randomized clinical trial. *Drug Des Devel Ther* 2023; **17**: 3563–3570, doi:10.2147/dddt.S427291.

157. Ghazaly, H. F., *et al.* A pre-anesthetic bolus of ketamine versus dexmedetomidine for prevention of postoperative delirium in elderly patients undergoing emergency surgery: a randomized, double-blinded, placebo-controlled study. *BMC Anesthesiol* 2023; **23**: 407, doi:10.1186/s12871-023-02367-8.

158. Zhang, D., *et al.* Melatonin or its analogs as premedication to prevent emergence agitation in children: a systematic review and meta-analysis. *BMC Anesthesiol* 2023; **23**, 392, doi:10.1186/s12871-023-02356-x.

159. Youn, Y. C. *et al.* Rivastigmine patch reduces the incidence of postoperative delirium in older patients with cognitive impairment. *Int J Geriatr Psychiatry* 2016; **32**: 1079–1084, doi:10.1002/gps.4569.

160. Marcantonio, E. R., *et al.* Pilot randomized trial of donepezil hydrochloride for delirium after hip fracture. *J Am Geriatr Soc* 2011; **59** Suppl 2: S282–288, doi:10.1111/j.1532-5415.2011.03691.x.

161. Overshott, R., *et al.* Cholinesterase inhibitors for delirium. *Cochrane Database System Rev* 2008; Cd005317, doi:10.1002/14651858.CD005317.pub2.

162. Sampson, E. L. *et al.* A randomized, double-blind, placebo-controlled trial of donepezil hydrochloride (Aricept) for reducing the incidence of postoperative delirium after elective total hip replacement. *Int J Geriatr Psychiatry* 2007; **22**: 343–349, doi:10.1002/gps.1679.

163. Liptzin, B., *et al.* Donepezil in the prevention and treatment of post-surgical delirium. *Am J Geriatr Psychiatry* 2005; **13**: 1100–1106, doi:10.1176/appi.ajgp.13.12.1100.

164. Lieberman, O. J., *et al.* Donepezil treatment is associated with improved outcomes in critically ill dementia patients via a reduction in delirium. *Alzheimers Dement* 2023; **19**: 1742–1751, doi:10.1002/alz.12807.

165. Asleson, D. R. *et al.* Melatonin for delirium prevention in acute medically ill, and perioperative geriatric patients. *Aging Medicine (Milton (N.S.W))* 2020; **3**: 132–137, doi:10.1002/agm2.12112.

166. Campbell, A. M. *et al.* Melatonin for the prevention of postoperative delirium in older adults: a systematic review and meta-analysis. *BMC Geriat* 2019; **19**: 272, doi:10.1186/s12877-019-1297-6.

167. Ford, A. H. *et al.* The healthy heart-mind trial: Randomized controlled trial of melatonin for prevention of delirium. *Journal of the American Geriatrics Society* 2020; **68**: 112–119, doi:10.1111/jgs.16162.

168. Niyogi, S. G., *et al.* Melatonin and melatonin agonists for prevention of delirium in the cardiac surgical ICU: A Meta-analysis. *Indian J Crit Care Med* 2023; **27**: 837–844, doi:10.5005/jp-journals-10071-24571.

169. Dobry, P., *et al.* Does melatonin decrease the use of as-needed antipsychotics or benzodiazepines in noncritically ill hospitalized patients? A multicenter retrospective cohort study. *J Integr Complement Med*, 2023; doi:10.1089/jicm.2023.0170.

170. Singla, L., *et al.* Oral melatonin as part of multimodal anxiolysis decreases emergence delirium in children whereas midazolam does not: A randomised, double-blind, placebo-controlled study. *Eur J Anaesthesiol* 2021; **38**: 1130–1137, doi:10.1097/eja.0000000000001561.

171. Oh, E. S. *et al.* Effects of ramelteon on the prevention of postoperative delirium in older patients undergoing orthopedic surgery: The RECOVER randomized controlled trial. *Am J Geriatr Psychiatry* 2020 [Epub ahead of print], doi:10.1016/j.jagp.2020.05.006.

172. Hatta, K. *et al.* Preventive effects of ramelteon on delirium: a randomized placebo-controlled trial. *JAMA Psychiatry* 2014; **71**: 397–403, doi:10.1001/jamapsychiatry.2013.3320.

173. Jaiswal, S. J. *et al.* Ramelteon for prevention of postoperative delirium: A randomized controlled trial in patients undergoing elective pulmonary thromboendarterectomy. *Crit Care Med* 2019; **47**: 1751–1758, doi:10.1097/ccm.0000000000004004.

174. Ikeuchi, S. *et al.* Efficacy of combined use of Suvorexant and Ramelteon in preventing postoperative delirium: A retrospective comparative study. *J Pharm Health Care Sci* 2023; **9**: 42, doi:10.1186/s40780-023-00311-z.

175. Adams, A. D., *et al.* The role of suvorexant in the prevention of delirium during acute hospitalization: A systematic review. *J Crit Care* 2020; **59**: 1–5, doi:10.1016/j.jcrc.2020.05.006.

176. Tian, Y., *et al.* Suvorexant with or without ramelteon to prevent delirium: a systematic review and meta-analysis. *Psychogeriatrics* 2022; **22**: 259–268, doi:10.1111/psyg.12792.

177. Lu, Y. *et al.* Promoting sleep and circadian health may prevent postoperative delirium: A systematic review and meta-analysis of randomized clinical trials. *Sleep Medicine Reviews* 2019; **48**: 101207, doi:10.1016/j.smrv.2019.08.001.

178. Dal-Pizzol, F. *et al.* Prophylactic minocycline for delirium in critically ill patients: a randomized controlled trial. *Chest* 2023; doi:10.1016/j.chest.2023.11.041.

179. Duprey, M. S. *et al.* Association between perioperative medication use and postoperative delirium and cognition in older adults undergoing elective noncardiac surgery. *Anesth Analg* 2022; **134**: 1154–1163, doi:10.1213/ane.0000000000005959.

180. Swarbrick, C. J. *et al.* Evidence-based strategies to reduce the incidence of postoperative delirium: a narrative review. *Anaesthesia* 2022; **77** Suppl 1: 92–101, doi:10.1111/anae.15607.

181. Tachibana, M. *et al.* Factors associated with the severity of delirium. *Hum Psychopharmacol* 2021; **36**: e2787, doi:10.1002/hup.2787.

182. Salvi, F. *et al.* Non-pharmacological approaches in the prevention of delirium. *Eur Geriatr Med* **11**: 71–81, doi:10.1007/s41999-019-00260-7.

183. Yuksel, J. M., *et al.* Optimal injectable haloperidol dose assessment in the older hospitalized inpatient. *Ann Pharmacother* 2023; **57**: 662–668, doi:10.1177/10600280221124615.

184. Wang, E. H. Z., *et al.* Haloperidol dosing strategies in the treatment of delirium in the critically-ill. *Neurocritical Care* 2012; **16**: 170–183, doi:10.1007/s12028-011-9643-3.

185. Liu, S. B. *et al.* Olanzapine for the treatment of ICU delirium: A systematic review and meta-analysis. *Ther Adv Psychopharmacol* 2023; **13**: 20451253231152113, doi:10.1177/20451253231152113.

186. Kirino, E. Use of aripiprazole for delirium in the elderly: a short review. *Psychogeriatrics* 2015; **15**: 75–84, doi:10.1111/psyg.12088.

187. Agar, M. R. *et al.* Efficacy of oral risperidone, haloperidol, or placebo for symptoms of delirium among patients in palliative care: A randomized clinical trial. *JAMA Internal Medicine* 2017; **177**: 34–42, doi:10.1001/jamainternmed.2016.7491.

End of Life Care

CONTENTS

INTRODUCTION

As patients approach the end of life, management of their psychiatric medication can become more complex. Reasons for this may include loss of a reliable oral route, changes in drug metabolism due to organ failure and weight loss, addition of new medications to treat progressing physical symptoms, and patient preferences regarding what is

The Maudsley® Prescribing Guidelines for Mental Health Conditions in Physical Illness, First Edition.
Siobhan Gee and David M. Taylor.
© 2025 John Wiley & Sons Ltd. Published 2025 by John Wiley & Sons Ltd.

important to them in the last days of life (e.g. they may wish to be at home or in a setting that feels 'non-medical'). Blood tests or use of the intravenous route are often not felt to be appropriate in the end of life setting, and may become practically difficult. Decisions about medication may be different depending on the expected prognosis of the condition, but the timescale is not always straightforward to predict, particularly in patients with conditions other than cancer. For many patients, continuation of psychiatric medication may be desirable, as withdrawal symptoms and/or relapse of the psychiatric illness bring unwelcome complications in the end stages of life.

Patients who are taking psychiatric medication and have been given a life-limiting diagnosis should be given the opportunity to express their own priorities in relation to their medication and make an advance plan for their wishes as their illness progresses with support from relevant clinical teams. Patients who have had severe mental illness may have a strong preference to avoid risking a relapse of this illness. They will benefit from both psychiatric and palliative care input to plan ways to minimise this risk.

ANTIDEPRESSANTS

Stopping antidepressants

Withdrawal symptoms are likely to occur on cessation of long-term antidepressants. These can occur within days. The level of risk is influenced by several factors. These include duration of use (longer durations being worse), past experience of withdrawal symptoms, dose (higher doses are worse), and the characteristics of the drug itself[1]. Drugs with shorter half-lives, no active metabolites, and high binding affinities for the central serotonin transporter may be more problematic[1].

Stopping drugs that are considered to have a low risk of causing withdrawal symptoms is unlikely to cause problems within the last weeks of life. Other drugs may need to be continued. Where drugs such as amitriptyline are being used in low doses for pain, they can usually be stopped abruptly.

Low risk of withdrawal symptoms[1]	Agomelatine Fluoxetine Milnacipran Trimipramine Doxepin Dosulepin
Medium risk of withdrawal symptoms[1]	Citalopram Escitalopram Sertraline Vortioxetine Nortriptyline Clomipramine Lofepramine
High risk of withdrawal symptoms[1]	Venlafaxine Duloxetine Paroxetine Phenelzine Moclobemide Amitriptyline Imipramine Mirtazapine

If the ability to safely swallow tablets is lost, consider switching to a liquid or orodispersible preparation (see chapter 3 for a list of options available at the time of writing in the UK market). Formulations such as citalopram oral drops require small volumes to deliver therapeutic doses (20mg is contained in 10 drops, approximately 0.5ml). It may not be necessary to replace the long-standing prescription exactly (same drug, same dose) to mitigate uncomfortable withdrawal symptoms. Where the drug required is not available either in liquid or orodispersible form, and crushing tablets is not an option, use an appropriate formulation of another drug in the same class in the first instance. If this is not possible, use fluoxetine or citalopram drops either orally or sublingually. For example, anecdotal success has been reported using fluoxetine liquid sublingually to prevent venlafaxine withdrawal symptoms.

Treating depression at the end of life

A new presentation of depressive symptoms may be very difficult to separate from physical and psychological aspects of approaching the end of life, and patients will benefit from skilled assessment and psychological support from palliative care teams as a first-line intervention.

Drug management of depression may be more important if a patient has an established recurrent depressive disorder and appears to be relapsing, in which case prompt input from both psychiatric and palliative care teams will be important to advise on management. Speed of response is clearly important, but do not rule out using conventional oral antidepressants, which can be effective in this population[2]. If the prognosis is less than a few weeks then there may not be sufficient time for a response to oral antidepressants. Further, the oral route is often unavailable in the last week of life. ECT is an effective treatment for depression but has challenges in the palliative care setting in terms of where this can be delivered and lack of reliable intravenous access; it may be an option in particular circumstances (e.g. history of good response to ECT) if expert input from both psychiatric and palliative care teams is available.

Intravenous (IV) administration of antidepressants has been used to speed response to oral drugs, but robust data to support the effectiveness of this strategy are lacking. It is also usual practice to avoid giving drugs intravenously in the last weeks of life, partly because it can be logistically difficult to manage cannulas in home environments, and because it can become difficult to cannulate patients towards the end of life and repeated attempts to do so may be unacceptably distressing. Further, very few antidepressants are available commercially in IV formulations. IV clomipramine[3] is available in Italy, and IV citalopram[4] can be obtained from Germany. Importing these formulations to other countries can take several weeks. See chapter 13 on non-oral formulations for more information. Note also that the increased speed of onset compared with oral formulations is presumed to be a result of higher plasma concentrations, which may not be tolerated in patients at the end of life. Alternative drug options for depression that can provide rapid symptom relief are psychostimulants and ketamine.

Psychostimulants

Methylphenidate[5] (5–30mg/day) and dexamphetamine[6] (2.5–20mg/day), either as monotherapy or in combination with a conventional antidepressant, can be beneficial within hours for mood, fatigue, and pain. Evidence is limited and response is not guaranteed[7].

Ketamine

Ketamine is licensed as an anaesthetic agent and is also commonly used as an adjuvant in cancer pain. An N-methyl-D-aspartate channel blocker, ketamine has a novel mechanism of action in the treatment of depression and also a varied method of delivery. Ketamine can be given IV, intramuscularly (IM), subcutaneously (SC), orally, or sublingually (SL), and can bring about rapid resolution of depressive symptoms (within hours).

IV administration of ketamine is more effective than administration by other routes, so where possible it should be given IV at initiation and switched to an alternative route after response is established (SC, SL, oral)[8]. In patients at the end of life, the IV route may not be practical and so SC administration can be used from the start. Doses should start at 0.5mg/kg (or 0.25mg/kg in elderly or very frail patients), given as an IV infusion over 40 minutes, or as a SC or IM bolus, or SL (hold ketamine solution under the tongue for 5 minutes, or use SL ketamine lozenges)[9]. If there is no response, increase the dose in 0.5mg increments to a maximum of 1mg/kg (1.5mg/kg for SL route). IV, SC, and IM doses should be given once or twice a week, or every 1–3 days for SL. Once response is established, dosing frequency of IV, IM, or SC administration can be reduced.

ANTIPSYCHOTICS

The risk of withdrawing antipsychotics is relapse of the psychiatric disorder and withdrawal symptoms (including rebound psychosis). If oral administration becomes unreliable, consider using liquid or orodispersible preparations. Alternative routes are IM, IV, or SC, described below.

Unless directly contraindicated, it is usually advisable to continue clozapine at the end of life because of the risk of relapse, rebound psychosis, or withdrawal catatonia on sudden cessation. It should not be necessary to continue FBC monitoring.

Intramuscular

Some antipsychotics are available as short-acting IM formulations (olanzapine, aripiprazole, haloperidol, clozapine). These may be useful for infrequent or short-term use, but less desirable if regular administration is necessary. Use of depot or long-acting injectable preparations may be beneficial, avoiding oral or daily IM administration. For patients who are already established on long-acting injections, it is unlikely to be necessary to give a dose in the last few weeks of life if administration has been consistent up to that point, since plasma concentrations will remain for some time with a gradual natural taper over many months.

Intravenous

Haloperidol and droperidol

Haloperidol can be given IV, although the manufacturer recommends continuous cardiac monitoring for QTc interval prolongation and ventricular arrhythmia if this route is used. At the end of life, the need for cardiac monitoring is questionable. Droperidol can also be given IV, and is licensed for prevention and treatment of postoperative nausea and vomiting via this route, albeit in much smaller doses than would be required for management of psychosis.

Olanzapine

Olanzapine has been given as an IV bolus using the short-acting IM product. Published data describe use for the management of agitation, often in emergency departments[10,11], and for treatment of psychosis or delirium in medically ill patients[12,13]. Similarly to the IM route, peak plasma concentrations are likely to be considerably higher than seen with the oral formulation, so doses should be initially low (1.25–2.5mg) and increased if necessary to a maximum of 10mg as a single dose. Doses may be repeated over a 24h period if needed, to a maximum of 20mg. Adverse effects appear to be mainly hypotension and bradycardia. Respiratory complications are described in some patients, but these are not all clearly attributed to olanzapine[14], and rates are similar with IM administration[15]. If parenteral benzodiazepines are given concurrently with IV olanzapine, monitor for cardiorespiratory depression, a complication reported (albeit not consistently) with the combination of IM olanzapine and IM benzodiazepines[16]. Olanzapine is also antiemetic, a feature that may be of particular use in this population[17].

Aripiprazole

Use of aripiprazole IV has not been described outside pharmacokinetic trials using infusions that are not commercially available[18].

Subcutaneous

Haloperidol and levomepromazine

Haloperidol and levomepromazine are commonly delivered via SC syringe drivers in palliative care for management of nausea and vomiting, agitation, and delirium. Typical doses are much lower than those that would usually be required for management of psychosis, and tolerability of higher doses may be difficult. Other antipsychotics (depot, IM, or oral if this route is still available) for the treatment of psychosis can be used in addition to low-dose antipsychotics delivered in syringe drivers without undue concern about combining drugs.

Risperidone

A once-monthly SC administered formulation of risperidone is licensed in the USA (Uzedy™)[19].

Olanzapine

SC administration of olanzapine is described in the literature either for use in delirium[20] or managing psychosis at the end of life[21]. The short-acting IM formulation can be given SC as a bolus injection. A maximum single dose of 10mg is recommended due to higher peak plasma concentrations achieved using parenteral olanzapine compared with oral. Doses can be given twice[21], or even three times[20] daily if required. Continuous SC infusion over 24 h using a syringe driver has also been described[21]. Both methods of administration appear to be well tolerated. Like many other end of life care drugs, olanzapine is a weak acid, but compatibility with other drugs in a syringe driver is unknown. Seek expert advice in the preparation of test mixes and observe carefully.

MOOD STABILISERS

If oral administration with tablets or capsules becomes challenging, most mood stabilisers are available in liquid preparations. If swallowing is not possible, or enteral absorption is problematic, asenapine (an antipsychotic with mood-stabilising activity, particularly antimanic) may be particularly useful, as it is absorbed in the buccal cavity. Olanzapine may also be used, and can be given in a variety of ways as described above. The antiepileptic drug levetiracetam is frequently used for seizure control at the end of life, and can be given via syringe driver. There are very limited data suggesting some possible efficacy for mania in bipolar disorder (not depression)[22].

Sodium valproate

Sodium valproate comes in a wide variety of formulations, including granules, which can be sprinkled onto soft foods. It is available as an IV injection that can be given directly, or by infusion. It can also be given via SC infusion. SC doses described in the literature (largely for seizure control) range from 500 to 2500mg/day[23].

Lithium

There is a risk of toxicity of lithium if fluid intake is limited and/or if renal function deteriorates. Venepuncture to monitor plasma concentrations may not be desirable at the end of life. However, given the risk of relapse (particularly if cessation is abrupt[24]), continuation of lithium when the prognosis is weeks to months is preferable. Consider reducing the dose if fluid intake or renal function is declining, and observe the patient for signs of toxicity.

References

1. Horowitz, M. A., Framer, A., Hengartner, M. P., Sørensen, A. & Taylor, D. Estimating risk of antidepressant withdrawal from a review of published data. *CNS Drugs* 2023; 37: 143–157, doi:10.1007/s40263-022-00960-y.

2. Perusinghe, M., Chen, K. Y. & McDermott, B. Evidence-based management of depression in palliative care: a systematic review. *J Palliat Med* 2021; 24: 767–781, doi:10.1089/jpm.2020.0659.

3. Pollock, B. G., Perel, J. M., Nathan, R. S. & Kupfer, D. J. Acute antidepressant effect following pulse loading with intravenous and oral clomipramine. *Arch Gen Psychiatry* 1989; 46: 29–35, doi:10.1001/archpsyc.1989.01810010031005.

4. Kasper, S. & Müller-Spahn, F. Intravenous antidepressant treatment: focus on citalopram. *Eur Arch Psychiatry Clin Neurosci* 2002; 252: 105–109, doi:10.1007/s00406-002-0363-8.

5. Centeno, C. et al. Multicentre, double-blind, randomised placebo-controlled clinical trial on the efficacy of methylphenidate on depressive symptoms in advanced cancer patients. *BMJ Support Palliat Care* 2012; 2: 328–333, doi:10.1136/bmjspcare-2011-000093.

6. Candy, B., Jones, L., Williams, R., Tookman, A. & King, M. in *Cochrane Database of Systematic Reviews* (2008).

7. Sullivan, D. R., Mongoue-Tchokote, S., Mori, M., Goy, E. & Ganzini, L. Randomized, double-blind, placebo-controlled study of methylphenidate for the treatment of depression in SSRI-treated cancer patients receiving palliative care. *Psychooncology* 2017; **26**: 1763–1769, doi:10.1002/pon.4220.

8. Goldman, N., Frankenthaler, M. & Klepacz, L. The efficacy of ketamine in the palliative care setting: a comprehensive review of the literature. *J Palliat Med* 2019; **22**: 1154–1161, doi:10.1089/jpm.2018.0627.

9. Taylor, D. M., Barnes, T. R. E. & Young, A. H. *The Maudsley® Prescribing Guidelines in Psychiatry.* 14 edn, (Wiley Blackwell, 2021).

10. Khorassani, F. & Saad, M. Intravenous olanzapine for the management of agitation: review of the literature. *Annals of Pharmacotherapy* 2019; **53**: 853–859, doi:10.1177/1060028019831634.

11. Chan, E. W. et al. Intravenous droperidol or olanzapine as an adjunct to midazolam for the acutely agitated patient: a multicenter, randomized, double-blind, placebo-controlled clinical trial. *Ann Emerg Med* 2013; **61**: 72–81, doi:10.1016/j.annemergmed.2012.07.118.

12. Hunt, N. F., McLaughlin, K. C., Kovacevic, M. P., Lupi, K. E. & Dube, K. M. Safety of Intravenous olanzapine administration at a tertiary academic medical center. *Ann Pharmacother* 2021; **55**: 1127–1133, doi:10.1177/1060028020988734.

13. Lorenzo, M. P., Burgess, J. & Darko, W. Intravenous olanzapine in a critically ill patient: an evolving route of administration. *Hosp Pharm* 2020; **55**: 108–111, doi:10.1177/0018578718823484.

14. Martel, M. L., Klein, L. R., Rivard, R. L. & Cole, J. B. A large retrospective cohort of patients receiving intravenous olanzapine in the emergency department. *Acad Emerg Med* 2016; **23**: 29–35, doi:10.1111/acem.12842.

15. Cole, J. B. et al. A prospective observational study of patients receiving intravenous and intramuscular olanzapine in the emergency department. *Ann Emerg Med* 2017; **69**: 327–336.e322, doi:10.1016/j.annemergmed.2016.08.008.

16. Williams, A. M. Coadministration of intramuscular olanzapine and benzodiazepines in agitated patients with mental illness. *Ment Health Clin* 2018; **8**: 208–213, doi:10.9740/mhc.2018.09.208.

17. Zhang, X. L. & Ying, J. E. Olanzapine for the prevention and treatment of chemotherapy-induced nausea and vomiting: a review to identify the best way to administer the drug. *Curr Oncol* 2022; **29**: 8235–8243, doi:10.3390/curroncol29110650.

18. Boulton, D. W. et al. Pharmacokinetics and tolerability of intramuscular, oral and intravenous aripiprazole in healthy subjects and in patients with schizophrenia. *Clin Pharmacokinet* 2008; **47**: 475–485, doi:10.2165/00003088-200847070-00004.

19. Tchobaniouk, L. V. et al. Once-monthly subcutaneously administered risperidone in the treatment of schizophrenia: patient considerations. *Patient Prefer Adherence* 2019; **13**: 2233–2241, doi:10.2147/ppa.S192418.

20. Elsayem, A. et al. Subcutaneous olanzapine for hyperactive or mixed delirium in patients with advanced cancer: a preliminary study. *J Pain Symptom Manage* 2010; **40**: 774–782, doi:10.1016/j.jpainsymman.2010.02.017.

21. Hindmarsh, J., Huggin, A., Belfonte, A., Lee, M. & Pickard, J. Subcutaneous olanzapine at the end of life in a patient with schizophrenia and dysphagia. *Palliat Med Rep* 2020; **1**: 72–75, doi:10.1089/pmr.2020.0039.

22. Kishi, T. et al. Levetiracetam for bipolar disorder: Consideration from a systematic review. *Bipolar Disord* 2022; **24**: 834–835, doi:10.1111/bdi.13255.

23. Kondasinghe, J. S., Look, M. L., Moffat, P. & Bradley, K. Subcutaneous levetiracetam and sodium valproate use in palliative care patients. *J Pain Palliat Care Pharmacother* 2022; **36**: 228–232, doi:10.1080/15360288.2022.2107145.

24. Cavanagh, J., Smyth, R. & Goodwin, G. M. Relapse into mania or depression following lithium discontinuation: a 7-year follow-up. *Acta Psychiatr Scand* 2004 **109**: 91–95, doi:10.1046/j.1600-0447.2003.00274.x.

Sickle Cell Disease

CONTENTS

INTRODUCTION

Sickle cell disease is an autosomal recessive inherited disorder, which is characterised by chronic anaemia, painful vaso-occlusive events, and end-organ damage[1]. It affects millions of people globally and is associated with shortened life expectancy and reduced quality of life[1].

In a survey spanning 16 countries, across six geographical regions, 39% of patients reported depression, and 38% anxiety. Prevalence estimates for depression in empirical studies vary widely, ranging from 0 to 85%[2]. Patients with comorbid depression have more frequent painful episodes[3] and more hospitalisations per year than those without[4]. Those with severe sickle cell disease are at higher risk of depression, owing to frequent painful and damaging crises, socioeconomic stress, and other psychological and social stressors[4]. Comparative data are not available for other serious mental illnesses.

The Maudsley® Prescribing Guidelines for Mental Health Conditions in Physical Illness, First Edition.
Siobhan Gee and David M. Taylor.
© 2025 John Wiley & Sons Ltd. Published 2025 by John Wiley & Sons Ltd.

ANTIDEPRESSANTS

There are no direct contraindications for any particular antidepressant regimen in people with sickle cell disease, nor are there data to support the efficacy of one drug over another. TCAs and SNRIs may appear attractive because of their role in management of neuropathic pain, but there are no data supporting use specifically in the vaso-occlusive pain experienced in sickle cell disease (limited data in children do not show superiority over SSRIs[5]). Effective treatment of the depressive symptoms, using whichever antidepressant is necessary to achieve response, is more important. Do not use trazodone in men – see section on priapism.

ANTIPSYCHOTICS

Sickle cell disease increases the risk of venous thromboembolism[6]. Antipsychotics, particularly at the start of treatment, are also associated with an increased risk of thrombus. The absolute risk is small (an excess of four extra cases of venous thromboembolism per 10,000 patients over a year for people of all ages prescribed an antipsychotic, and 10 extra cases for patients aged 65 and over[7]), but if antipsychotics can be avoided (if another drug, or non-drug measure can be used), do so. Otherwise, there are no direct contraindications to antipsychotics in sickle cell disease, but avoid risperidone in men – see section on priapism.

MOOD STABILISERS

There is no contraindication to any of the mood-stabilising antiepileptics or lithium in sickle cell disease. Patients taking non-steroidal anti-inflammatory drugs (NSAIDs) are at risk of lithium toxicity due to a reduction in prostaglandins decreasing renal blood flow, impairing lithium excretion. Adjustment of lithium doses to account for the interaction is possible for patients who take NSAIDs continuously, but intermittent use makes this difficult.

PRIAPISM

Men with sickle cell disease are at increased risk of priapism[8]. Antipsychotics account for about 50% of case of drug-induced priapism[9], with a presumed pathophysiology of peripheral alpha-1 adrenergic blockade interfering with sympathetic control of penile detumescence[9]. Avoid drugs with greater peripheral alpha-adrenergic affinity, such as chlorpromazine and risperidone[10,11], particularly for patients who take other alpha-blocking drugs (including illicit substances such as cocaine[12]). Adding other drugs that increase the plasma concentration of the alpha-blocking medication may also increase the risk of priapism[13-15].

Of the antidepressants, trazodone is associated with priapism (it is also an alpha-blocker) and should thus be avoided[16].

DRUG INTERACTIONS

Case reports describe reductions in carbamazepine and valproate serum concentrations by hydroxycarbamide. Monitor plasma concentrations.

References

1. Osunkwo, I., *et al.* Impact of sickle cell disease on patients' daily lives, symptoms reported, and disease management strategies: Results from the international Sickle Cell World Assessment Survey (SWAY). *Am J Hematol* 2021; **96**: 404–417, doi:10.1002/ajh.26063.

2. Oudin Doglioni, D., *et al.* Depression in adults with sickle cell disease: a systematic review of the methodological issues in assessing prevalence of depression. *BMC Psychol* 2021; **9**: 54, doi:10.1186/s40359-021-00543-4.

3. Harris, K. M., *et al.* Examining mental health, education, employment, and pain in sickle cell disease. *JAMA Network Open* 2023; **6**: e2314070–e2314070, doi:10.1001/jamanetworkopen.2023.14070.

4. Jonassaint, C. R., *et al.* A systematic review of the association between depression and health care utilization in children and adults with sickle cell disease. *Br J Haematol* 2016; **174**: 136–147, doi:10.1111/bjh.14023.

5. Jerrell, J. M., Tripathi, A. & Stallworth, J. R. Pain management in children and adolescents with sickle cell disease. *Am J Hematol* 2011; **86**: 82–84, doi:10.1002/ajh.21873.

6. Noubiap, J. J. *et al.* Sickle cell disease, sickle trait and the risk for venous thromboembolism: a systematic review and meta-analysis. *Thrombosis J* 2018; **16**, 27, doi:10.1186/s12959-018-0179-z.

7. Parker, C., *et al.* Antipsychotic drugs and risk of venous thromboembolism: nested case-control study. *BMJ* 2010; **341**, c4245, doi:10.1136/bmj.c4245.

8. Hwang, T., *et al.* A review of antipsychotics and priapism. *Sex Med Rev* 2021; **9**: 464–471, doi: https://doi.org/10.1016/j.sxmr.2020.10.003.

9. Scherzer, N. D., *et al.* Unintended consequences: a review of pharmacologically-induced priapism. *Sex Med Rev* 2019; **7**: 283–292, doi:10.1016/j.sxmr.2018.09.002.

10. Compton, M. T. *et al.* Priapism associated with conventional and atypical antipsychotic medications: a review. *J Clin Psychiatry* 2001; **62**: 362–366, doi:10.4088/jcp.v62n0510.

11. Andersohn, F., *et al.* Priapism associated with antipsychotics: role of α1 adrenoceptor affinity. *J Clin Psychopharmacology* 2010; **30**: 68–71, doi:10.1097/JCP.0b013e3181c8273d.

12. Koirala, S., *et al.* Priapism and risperidone. *South Med J* 2009; **102**: 1266–1268, doi:10.1097/SMJ.0b013e3181c04775.

13. Geraci, M. J., *et al.* Antipsychotic-induced priapism in an HIV patient: a cytochrome P450-mediated drug interaction. *Inter J Emer Med* 2010; **3**: 81–84.

14. Yang, P. *et al.* Occurrence of priapism with risperidone-paroxetine combination in an autistic child. *J Child Adol Psychopharmacol* 2004; **14**: 342.

15. Seger, A. *et al.* Priapism associated with polypharmacy. *J Clin Psychiatry* 2001; **62**: 128, doi:10.4088/jcp.v62n0210d.

16. Rezaee, M. E. *et al.* Are we overstating the risk of priapism with oral phosphodiesterase type 5 inhibitors? *J Sex Med* 2020; **17**, 1579–1582, doi:10.1016/j.jsxm.2020.05.019.

Chapter 10

Corticosteroid-induced Psychiatric Adverse Effects

CONTENTS

INTRODUCTION

Glucocorticoids and mineralocorticoids are steroid hormones, secreted predominantly by the adrenal glands. Glucocorticoids include corticosterone and cortisol, and mineralocorticoids include aldosterone. Together, they are termed *corticosteroids*. Glucocorticoids regulate metabolic activity, immune function, and behaviour[1]. Mineralocorticoids increase sodium resorption in the kidneys, salivary glands, and intestine[1]. Synthetic versions of these hormones are modified to enhance anti-inflammatory effects and extend biological duration of action. These synthetic

The Maudsley® Prescribing Guidelines for Mental Health Conditions in Physical Illness, First Edition.
Siobhan Gee and David M. Taylor.
© 2025 John Wiley & Sons Ltd. Published 2025 by John Wiley & Sons Ltd.

chemicals may possess predominantly glucocorticoid (e.g. prednisolone, triamcinolone, methylprednisolone, dexamethasone) or mineralocorticoid properties (e.g. fludrocortisone). Their immune-suppressing and anti-inflammatory properties are used in a wide range of clinical situations, including allergy, rheumatic disease, gastrointestinal disorders, ophthalmic conditions, dermatological conditions, asthma, chronic obstructive pulmonary disease, systemic lupus erythematosus, cancer, and to avoid transplant rejection.

Psychiatric effects of corticosteroids

Since their introduction to clinical use in the 1950s, physical and neuropsychiatric adverse effects of corticosteroids have been recorded in both acute and chronic use. Psychiatric symptoms include depression, anxiety, psychosis, and mania. It is suggested that short-term use of corticosteroids is more often associated with euphoria or mania, and depression occurs more frequently with long-term prescriptions[2]. This is consistent with the observation that depression is common in Cushing's disease, a disorder of chronic excess endogenous corticosteroid excess, occurring in more than 50% of patients[3]. Synthetic corticosteroids have the same effect. In one cohort study, more than half of patients taking prednisone had developed neuropsychiatric symptoms by 3 months of treatment[4]. A large UK database study found the incidence of neuropsychiatric outcomes overall to be 22.2 cases per 100 person-years for first-course treatments[5]. In this study, compared with people with the same underlying medical disease, those treated with glucocorticoids were almost twice as likely to develop depression, four times as likely to develop mania, and five times as likely to develop delirium. They were seven times as likely to attempt suicide.

The mechanism for neuropsychiatric effects of corticosteroids is not clear. Cortisol is released from the adrenal glands in response to stress[6] and regulated by a negative feedback system. Administration of exogenous corticosteroids activates pituitary glucocorticoid receptors, whilst suppressing adrenal cortisol secretion, depleting endogenous cortisol, and reducing stimulation at mineralocorticoid receptors. The resulting imbalance between glucocorticoid and mineralocorticoid receptor activation may underlie the neuropsychiatric effects of glucocorticoid treatment[6,7]. High cortisol levels also inhibit brain-derived neurotrophic factor, low levels of which may contribute to depression and anxiety[8].

RISK FACTORS

The risk of experiencing a neuropsychiatric adverse effect with corticosteroid treatment increases with dose[5], although the dose does not predict onset, severity, or type or duration of symptoms[2]. The widely cited Boston Collaborative Drug Surveillance Program[9] examined 718 medical inpatients who were initiated on prednisone. They found acute psychiatric reactions occurred in only 1.3% of patients taking less than 40mg prednisone per day, but this increased to 4.6% of patients at 40–80mg per day, and 18% at doses of more than 80mg. Drug–drug interactions that increase the effective dose of a steroid have the same effect, and steroid-induced psychosis has been described after addition of clarithromycin to prednisone[10]. (Clarithromycin inhibits CYP3A4 enzyme activity, the route of metabolism of prednisolone – the active metabolite of prednisone.)

The risk also increases with age[5,9,11] and with history of previous neuropsychiatric adverse effects when taking corticosteroid treatment[5]. In one study, the hazard ratio of having a recurrence of the same psychiatric side effects experienced on a prior course of glucocorticoids was 1.32[5] – a 32% increased risk above baseline for the same adverse effect recurring.

Whether having a history of psychiatric illness increases the risk of experiencing psychiatric adverse effects as a result of corticosteroid treatment is not entirely clear. Small studies have found no link[2,12–14] (or even an improvement in depression during corticosteroid treatment[15]). In contrast, a large primary care study found patients with a prior history of depression, mania, panic disorder, suicide attempt, or delirium (psychotic disorders were not included) were at increased risk of developing the same disorder when exposed to glucocorticoids[5]. The size of this study and associated statistical power lend it more weight than the earlier reports.

TIME OF ONSET

Neuropsychiatric adverse effects can occur at any time, from almost immediately after initiation of the corticosteroid to some time after treatment has stopped. Most reactions appear to occur within the first few weeks. A review of case reports found a median time to onset of 11.5 days, with 39% of adverse reactions occurring in the first week, 62% within 2 weeks, and 83% within 6 weeks of initiation[11].

Corticosteroid-induced psychiatric effects can also occur as a result of corticosteroid withdrawal. A UK primary care database study found that during withdrawal from 1–3 years of glucocorticoid treatment, incident rates of depression were 11.1 per 100 person-years[16]. Depression was more common in the withdrawal period than delirium (3.9 per 100 patient-years), mania (0.4), or panic disorder (0.4). Having a history of depression increased the risk of developing depression during glucocorticoid discontinuation. Age, sex, or time period of glucocorticoid exposure had no influence. Longer-acting glucocorticoids (dexamethasone, betamethasone, triamcinolone) conferred more risk than shorter-acting drugs (prednisolone, methylprednisolone). The authors suggest that management strategies in these scenarios should include assessment for adrenal insufficiency (a range of psychiatric presentations, including depression, anxiety, mania, psychosis, and cognitive impairment, have been associated with adrenal insufficiency[17]), and then reintroduction of the corticosteroid[18], followed presumably by a more gradual withdrawal.

Neuropsychiatric symptoms may even occur after cessation of treatment. The corticosteroids dexamethasone and betamethasone have long half-lives (up to 54h[19]) and as a result may accumulate. Psychosis has been reported days after the last dose was given[20].

MANAGEMENT

Dose reduction of the corticosteroid, and ideally cessation, is the preferable management strategy should psychiatric side effects occur[2]. In principle, short courses of corticosteroids (less than 3 weeks) can be stopped abruptly. Long-term corticosteroids must be withdrawn slowly to minimise the risk of adrenal insufficiency and crisis[21]. A tapering plan should be drawn up by the medical team prescribing the corticosteroid and the patient monitored for signs of relapse of the condition they were prescribed to treat.

If the corticosteroid cannot be reduced or stopped, then specific management of the psychiatric adverse effect(s) may be required. Management strategies are discussed below.

Depression

Depression is the most common neuropsychiatric adverse effect reported with long-term glucocorticoid treatment, with reported prevalence rates at two to three times those of the general population[5,22]. Women appear to be at higher risk[5].

There are many case reports describing successful use of SSRIs, SNRIs, and lithium in the treatment of corticosteroid-induced depression[2,19], but no controlled trials to direct selection of one drug over another. TCAs should be avoided, given the heightened risk of suicide in this population. ECT has been used in corticosteroid-induced psychotic depression[19]. Treatment should be chosen based on the patient's medical and psychiatric treatment history.

Psychosis

There are no data to guide antipsychotic selection in the management of corticosteroid-induced psychosis. Avoid initiating TCAs – as well as the risk in suicide, some case series suggest they may worsen corticosteroid-induced psychoses[13,23,24]. ECT has been used successfully in cases unresponsive to pharmacotherapy[11,25].

Mania

Several publications report hypomania or mania to be the most common acute psychiatric adverse effect with corticosteroid treatment[19]. Men are more likely to develop mania or delirium than depression when taking glucocorticoids[5].

Numerous case reports describe the successful management of corticosteroid-induced mania or hypomania with a range of drugs, including antipsychotics, mood stabilisers, benzodiazepines, and combinations of all of these[19]. A single open-label trial of the use of olanzapine in 12 patients with corticosteroid-induced mania or mixed symptoms found it to be effective and well tolerated[26]. There are insufficient data to support the selection of any pharmacological strategy over another. Carbamazepine should be avoided as its induction of CYP3A4 results in lower plasma concentrations of glucocorticoids.

PROGNOSIS

Psychiatric adverse effects with corticosteroids are reversible on stopping the treatment, but do not necessarily resolve immediately. A recent review of published case reports[27] suggested that the onset of recovery from corticosteroid-induced psychosis could be as soon as 24 hours after either treatment for the psychosis was started or the corticosteroid was stopped. On average, recovery occurred within a month. This finding is echoed by other reviews[28]. Patients who were able to discontinue the corticosteroid recovered more quickly than those who had treatment tapered or continued[27].

PROPHYLAXIS

Some data show a lower risk of corticosteroid-induced psychiatric adverse effects for patients who have had previous treatment with corticosteroids[5], probably because patients who have had psychiatric side effects before are less likely to be prescribed corticosteroids again. Given the important role corticosteroids can have in management of physical illnesses, it is therefore important to address any possible role for prevention in these cases, so patients are not unnecessarily excluded from effective treatments. 'Watchful waiting' is employed in some case reports[28], only prescribing treatment if adverse effects emerge. Close observation along with patient and carer education about the risk of psychiatric adverse effects is important.

There are many reports in the literature describing successful use of various pharmacological agents in the prevention of a range of psychiatric adverse effects in patients taking corticosteroids. Case reports and one small retrospective study have demonstrated successful use of various drugs, including lithium[29,30], chlorpromazine[31], and valproate[32] for the prevention of corticosteroid-induced psychosis, for example. Positive publication bias makes it impossible to assess the effectiveness of these strategies. Some authors suggest that patients with medical and neurological conditions that are themselves commonly associated with mood disorders should be particularly considered for prophylaxis (e.g. systemic lupus erythematosus, multiple sclerosis, epilepsy, Parkinson's disease, and Alzheimer's disease)[6]. There are no trial data to support routine pharmacological prophylaxis in these (or any other) populations, and so a better approach is a collaborative one with the patient, considering other risk factors (previous adverse effects with corticosteroids, previous psychiatric history, suicide risk, and so on).

SUMMARY

Neuropsychiatric adverse effects of corticosteroids	Mania, delirium, confusion are more common early in treatment. Depression is more common with chronic use; women are at higher risk. Withdrawal from steroids is also associated with adverse effects, particularly depression.
Risk factors	High doses. Older age. Previous psychiatric adverse effects when taking corticosteroids. Possibly pre-existing psychiatric diagnosis - data are conflicting.
Treatment	All options appear effective. No data are available to guide drug choice.
Prophylaxis	May be effective. No data are available to guide drug choice. There are insufficient data to support prophylaxis on the basis of pre-existing mental illness alone. May be considered for patients with multiple risk factors.

References

1. Taves, M. D., *et al*. Extra-adrenal glucocorticoids and mineralocorticoids: evidence for local synthesis, regulation, and function. *Am J Physiol Endocrinol Metab* 2011; **301**: E11–24, doi:10.1152/ajpendo.00100.2011.
2. Warrington, T. P. *et al*. Psychiatric adverse effects of corticosteroids. *Mayo Clinic Proceedings* 2006; **81**: 1361–1367, doi: https://doi.org/10.4065/81.10.1361.
3. Sonino, N., Fava, G. A., Raffi, A. R., Boscaro, M. & Fallo, F. Clinical correlates of major depression in Cushing's disease. *Psychopathology* 1998; **31**: 302–306, doi:10.1159/000029054.
4. Fardet, L. *et al*. Corticosteroid-induced clinical adverse events: frequency, risk factors and patient's opinion. *Br J Dermatology* 2007; **157**: 142–148, doi:10.1111/j.1365-2133.2007.07950.x.
5. Fardet, L., *et al*. Suicidal behavior and severe neuropsychiatric disorders following glucocorticoid therapy in primary care. *Am J Psychiatry* 2012; **169**: 491–497, doi:10.1176/appi.ajp.2011.11071009.
6. Judd, L. L. *et al*. Adverse consequences of glucocorticoid medication: psychological, cognitive, and behavioral effects. *Am J Psychiatry* 2014; **171**: 1045–1051, doi:10.1176/appi.ajp.2014.13091264.
7. de Kloet, E. R. *et al*. Stress and the brain: from adaptation to disease. *Nature Reviews Neuroscience* 2005; **6**: 463–475, doi:10.1038/nrn1683.
8. Duman, R. S. *et al*. A neurotrophic model for stress-related mood disorders. *Biol Psychiatry* 2006; **59**: 1116–1127, doi:10.1016/j.biopsych.2006.02.013.
9. Acute adverse reactions to prednisone in relation to dosage. *Clin Pharmacol Ther* 1972; **13**: 694–698, doi:10.1002/cpt1972135part1694.
10. Finkenbine, R. D. *et al*. Case of psychosis due to prednisone-clarithromycin interaction. *Gen Hosp Psychiatry* 1998; **20**: 325–326, doi:10.1016/s0163-8343(98)00032-2.
11. Lewis, D. A. *et al*. Steroid-induced psychiatric syndromes. A report of 14 cases and a review of the literature. *J Affect Disord* 1983; **5**: 319–332, doi:10.1016/0165-0327(83)90022-8.
12. Goolker, P. *et al*. Psychic effects of ACTH and cortisone. *Psychosom Med* 1953; **15**: 589–612; discussion, 612–583, doi:10.1097/00006842-195311000-00004.
13. Hall, R. C., *et al*. Presentation of the steroid psychoses. *J Nerv Ment Dis* 1979; **167**: 229–236, doi:10.1097/00005053-197904000-00006.
14. Lewis, A. *et al*. The psychiatric risk from corticotrophin and cortisone. *Lancet* 1954; **266**: 383–386, doi:10.1016/s0140-6736(54)90926-5.
15. Brown, E. S., *et al*. 3rd. Mood changes during prednisone bursts in outpatients with asthma. *J Clin Psychiatry* 2002; **22**: 55–61, doi:10.1097/00004714-200202000-00009.
16. Fardet, L., *et al*. Severe neuropsychiatric outcomes following discontinuation of long-term glucocorticoid therapy: a cohort study. *J Clin Psychiatry* 2013; **74**: e281–286, doi:10.4088/JCP.12m08034.
17. Perry, B. I. A psychiatric presentation of adrenal insufficiency: a case report. *Prim Care Companion CNS Disord* 2015; **17**, doi:10.4088/PCC.15l01819.
18. Hassanyeh, F., *et al*. Adrenocortical suppression presenting with agitated depression, morbid jealousy, and a dementia-like state. *Br J Psychiatry* 1991; **159**: 870–872, doi:10.1192/bjp.159.6.870.
19. Kenna, H. A., *et al*. Psychiatric complications of treatment with corticosteroids: review with case report. *Psych and Clin Neuro* 2011; 65.

20. Ferris, R. L. *et al.* Steroid psychosis after head and neck surgery: case report and review of the literature. *Otolaryngology–Head and Neck Surgery* 2003; **129**: 591–592, doi:10.1016/s0194-59980300717-4.

21. Baker, E. H. Is there a safe and effective way to wean patients off long-term glucocorticoids? *Br J Clin Pharmacol* 2020, doi:10.1111/bcp.14679.

22. Patten, S. B. Exogenous corticosteroids and major depression in the general population. *J Psychosom Res* 2000; **49**: 447–449, doi:10.1016/s0022-3999(00)00187-2.

23. Hall, R. C., *et al.* Tricyclic exacerbation of steroid psychosis. *J Nerv Ment Dis* 1978; **166**: 738–742.

24. Malinow, K. L. *et al.* Tricyclic precipitation of steroid psychosis. *Psychiatr Med* 1984; **2**: 351–354.

25. Davis, J. M. *et al.* Treatment of steroid psychoses. *Psychiatr Annals* 1992; **22**: 487–491, doi:10.3928/0048-5713-19920901-12.

26. Brown, E. S. *et al.* An open-label trial of olanzapine for corticosteroid-induced mood symptoms. *J Affect Disord* 2004; **83**: 277–281, doi:10.1016/j.jad.2004.07.001.

27. Huynh, G. *et al.* Pharmacological management of steroid-induced psychosis: a review of patient cases. *J Pharm Technol* 2021; **37**: 120–126, doi:10.1177/8755122520978534.

28. Ismail, M. F. *et al.* Steroid-induced mental disorders in cancer patients: a systematic review. *Future Oncology* 2017; **13**: 2719–2731.

29. Falk, W. E., *et al.* Lithium prophylaxis of corticotropin-induced psychosis. *JAMA* 1979; **241**: 1011–1012.

30. Goggans, F. C., *et al.* Lithium prophylaxis of prednisone psychosis: a case report. *J Clin Psychiatry* 1983; **44**: 111–112.

31. Bloch, M., *et al.* Chlorpromazine prophylaxis of steroid-induced psychosis. *Gen Hosp Psychiatry* 1994; **16**: 42–44, doi:10.1016/0163-8343(94)90086-8.

32. Abbas, A. *et al.* Valproate prophylaxis against steroid induced psychosis. *Can J Psychiatry* 1994; **39**: 188–189, doi:10.1177/070674379403900327.

CHAPTER 10

CONTENTS

GLAUCOMA AND SERIOUS MENTAL ILLNESS

'Glaucoma' describes a group of optic neuropathies that are characterised by progressive degeneration of retinal ganglion cells[1]. It affects at least 70 million people worldwide – the true number is likely to be higher, as the disease is frequently asymptomatic until severe[1]. Glaucoma is split into two categories: open-angle and angle-closure. The 'angle' refers to the angle between the iris and cornea. Primary open-angle glaucoma is most common (80% of cases). Angle-closure glaucoma is less common, and three-quarters of cases occur in women[2]. Prevalence of both conditions increases with age[2], possibly due to the increasing size of the lens[3].

The pathophysiology of glaucoma is not fully understood, but the principal issue is that of raised intraocular pressure causing retinal ganglion cell death. Under normal

The Maudsley® Prescribing Guidelines for Mental Health Conditions in Physical Illness, First Edition.
Siobhan Gee and David M. Taylor.
© 2025 John Wiley & Sons Ltd. Published 2025 by John Wiley & Sons Ltd.

circumstances, aqueous humour is secreted by the ciliary body of the eye and drained through two pathways – the trabecular mesh and uveoscleral outflow[1]. In open-angle glaucoma, the trabecular meshwork has increased resistance to aqueous flow, increasing the intraocular pressure. In angle-closure glaucoma, access to the drainage pathways is blocked[1]. Acute attacks of angle-closure glaucoma are precipitated by pupillary dilation causing the iris to bulge ('pupillary block'), acutely closing the angle between the iris and cornea, and are a medical emergency[3].

As with other chronic diseases and mental illness, there is an association between glaucoma and depression[4], anxiety[5], bipolar disorder[6], and schizophrenia[6]. Note that cardiovascular disease, a common comorbidity in serious mental illness, is also a major factor that influences the progression of glaucoma[7].

ANTIDEPRESSANTS

There are a variety of mechanisms through which antidepressants can both increase and decrease intraocular pressure. Serotonergic receptors are located in several different eye structures, and stimulation can variously reduce or enhance aqueous humour production and affect ciliary body blood flow[8]. Anything that is anticholinergic or noradrenergic carries a risk of causing or exacerbating acute angle-closure glaucoma in patients with pre-existing narrow angles, through pupillary dilation[9]. What this interplay between receptor effects means for clinical outcomes with individual drugs is not entirely clear.

TCAs and MAOIs

TCAs can precipitate acute angle-closure glaucoma attacks as their anticholinergic effects can cause pupil dilation. For the same reason, MAOIs are also a risk for angle-closure, although they have weaker anticholinergic effects. It is possible that the risk of an acute attack is additive if anticholinergic medicines are co-prescribed, so it is advisable to take account of the total prescriptions for the patient using a tool such as Medichec (Medichec.com).

The risk for patients with open-angle glaucoma is less clear, with at least one study showing no effect of TCAs on the risk of developing open-angle glaucoma[10].

SSRIs and SNRIs

Individual studies variously find no association between the use of SSRIs and either open-angle[10,11] or angle-closure glaucoma[11], and conversely an increased risk of angle-closure[12] or glaucoma as a whole[13]. Meta-analysis suggests that overall, there is no association between risk of glaucoma and use of serotonergic antidepressants[14] (but note that evidence is limited to case-control and cohort studies). One large case-control study in fact suggested a reduction in risk of open-angle glaucoma in patients taking selective serotonin reuptake inhibitors (SSRIs) (odds ratio 0.70) or serotonin-noradrenaline reuptake inhibitors (SNRIs) (odds ratio 0.71). This appeared to be an effect of the drugs themselves rather than depression as a diagnosis, and the study found a dose–response relationship, with higher doses being more protective than lower. This would give SSRI or SNRI users an overall 30% reduction in risk of open-angle glaucoma (there was no benefit observed for patients taking TCAs)[15]. By contrast, case reports describe increases in intraocular pressure with SSRIs, although these are few in number. Numerically more involve fluoxetine, paroxetine, and sertraline (compared with citalopram), possibly because of the relatively increased effects on noradrenaline uptake[16]. The reason for these conflicting conclusions is not clear; heterogeneity in study populations and study design may play a part.

SSRIs and SNRIs are undoubtedly less likely to cause attacks of acute angle-closure glaucoma than the TCAs or MAOIs, but they may not be entirely without risk. Case reports describe acute angle-closure attacks with various SSRIs and SNRIs[17]; it may be that increased levels of serotonin cause partial pupillary dilation and increased ciliary body blood low, increasing aqueous production[16]. Anticholinergic effects may also play a part. Noradrenergic and dopaminergic effects may lead to mydriasis and trigger acute angle closure, contributing to risk for SNRIs[18], vortioxetine, and SSRIs that also inhibit noradrenaline reuptake (e.g. paroxetine[16]).

Others

A large USA study found bupropion to be protective for open-angle glaucoma[10], with the beneficial effect accumulating with chronic use (0.6% reduced risk for each additional month of use, totalling a 21% reduced hazard over 1–2 years compared with non-users). Similarly to the data suggesting protection by SSRIs and SNRIs, this finding was independent of indication for bupropion. The authors propose that the anti-TNF action of bupropion may underpin this effect, and the finding is backed up at least one other, less well controlled study[19]. In contrast, a case-control study found that patients under 50 years of age taking bupropion had more than double the risk of acute angle-closure glaucoma compared with non-users (the effect was non-significant when older patients were included). Note, however, that acute angle-closure is a rare event, particularly in younger people, and the absolute risk remains small.

There are scant data relating to the risk of glaucoma with mirtazapine. The manufacturers caution of the possibility of pupillary dilation causing acute angle-closure, a concern that seems reasonable when considering the pharmacological action of mirtazapine, and this is described in one case report[20].

Agomelatine is the only antidepressant that appears to be definitively safe in acute angle-closure glaucoma and in open-angle glaucoma – in fact, it may be positively beneficial for glaucoma patients[21]. One small study (10 patients with open-angle glaucoma) found a significant reduction in intraocular pressure with agomelatine[22], possibly mediated through several different mechanisms (the influence of melatonin on adrenergic and dopaminergic pathways, down-regulation of carbonic anhydrase, modulation of glycosaminoglycan within trabecular meshwork, and protection of neurons from oxidative stress)[22,23]. Further studies are required to replicate this effect. One case report suggests reversal of SSRI-induced acute angle closure by agomelatine[24].

Recommendation

Open angle: bupropion, agomelatine, mirtazapine, SSRI (preferably citalopram).

Closed-angle: agomelatine. Avoid TCAs and bupropion. If an SSRI is required, avoid paroxetine, and ideally also sertraline or fluoxetine. Citalopram is preferred.

ANTIPSYCHOTICS

There is very little published literature describing any relationship between glaucoma and antipsychotics. One small study (28 patients) found raised intraocular pressure for patients taking ziprasidone, but not other antipsychotics[25]. This may be due to affinity of ziprasidone for serotonin receptors, but the finding needs replication. Otherwise, antipsychotics do not appear to be clearly associated with the risk of developing open angle glaucoma, but the impact of antipsychotic-induced cardiovascular disease on the progression of glaucoma may be important.

There are case reports describing an association of acute angle-closure glaucoma with various antipsychotics, including several with olanzapine[26-28] and one with aripiprazole[29], which may reflect anticholinergic activity. Note the likely additive risk if other anticholinergic medicines are used for the treatment of EPSEs alongside antipsychotics.

Recommendation

Open angle: no contraindications, avoid ziprasidone.

Closed angle: no contraindications, but prefer drugs with weaker anticholinergic effects (risperidone, sulpiride, amisulpride, haloperidol, lurasidone).

MOOD STABILISERS

Sodium valproate is suggested to be neuroprotective through antioxidative actions and inhibition of enzymes involved in apoptosis[30]. Neuroprotection of retinal ganglion cells may be helpful in the treatment of glaucoma, since it is retinal cell death that leads to sight loss. Animal studies suggest that valproate may be effective in the management of glaucoma by attenuating this cell death[31]. Clinical studies are limited to a single pilot study[32] showing improvement in visual acuity in 31 patients with advanced glaucoma.

Similarly, lithium exerts neuroprotective actions on retinal ganglion cells[33,34]. Demonstration of the clinical utility of this is so far limited to animal studies[35].

Topiramate, like other sulfa-based agents, can induce 'non-pupillary block' acute angle-closure glaucoma[36,37], and is also associated with an increased risk of developing glaucoma as a whole[38,39]. It should be avoided.

Carbamazepine and lamotrigine do not appear to be associated with glaucoma.

Recommendation

Do not use topiramate. Otherwise, no agent is contraindicated. Sodium valproate and lithium may be actively beneficial.

References

1. Weinreb, R. N., *et al.* The pathophysiology and treatment of glaucoma: A review. *Jama* 2014; **311**: 1901–1911, doi:10.1001/jama.2014.3192.

2. Day, A. C. *et al.* The prevalence of primary angle closure glaucoma in European derived populations: a systematic review. *Br J Ophthalmology* 2012; **96**: 1162–1167, doi:10.1136/bjophthalmol-2011-301189.

3. Khazaeni, B., *et al.* Acute closed angle glaucoma. *StatPearls* 2023; Jan 2. StatPearls Publishing.

4. Stamatiou, M. E., *et al.* Depression in glaucoma patients: A review of the literature. *Semin Ophthalmol* 2022; **37**,:29–35, doi:10.1080/0882 0538.2021.1903945.

5. Shin, D. Y., *et al.* The effect of anxiety and depression on progression of glaucoma. *Sci Rep* 2021; **11**: 1769, doi:10.1038/s41598-021-81512-0.

6. Liu, C. H. *et al.* Association of ocular diseases with schizophrenia, bipolar disorder, and major depressive disorder: a retrospective case-control, population-based study. *BMC Psychiatry* **20**: 486, doi:10.1186/s12888-020-02881-w (2020).

7. Chan, T. C. *et al.* Risk factors for rapid glaucoma disease progression. *Am J Ophthalmol* 2017; **180**: 151–157, doi:10.1016/j.ajo.2017.06.003.

8. Ciobanu, A. M. *et al.* Psychopharmacological treatment, intraocular pressure and the risk of glaucoma: a review of literature. *J Clin Med* **10**: doi:10.3390/jcm10132947 (2021).

9. Flores-Sánchez, B. C. *et al.* Acute angle closure glaucoma. *Br J Hosp Med (Lond)* 2019; **80**: C174–c179, doi:10.12968/hmed.2019.80.12.C174.

10. Stein, J. D. *et al.* Bupropion use and risk of open-angle glaucoma among enrollees in a large U.S. managed care network. *PLoS One* 2015; **10**: e0123682, doi:10.1371/journal.pone.0123682.

11. Chen, H. Y., *et al.* Long-term use of selective serotonin reuptake inhibitors and risk of glaucoma in depression patients. *Medicine (Baltimore)* 2015; **94**: e2041, doi:10.1097/md.0000000000002041.

12. Chen, H. Y., *et al.* Association of selective serotonin reuptake inhibitor use and acute angle-closure glaucoma. *J Clin Psychiatry* 2016; **77**: e692–696, doi:10.4088/JCP.15m10038.

13. Chen, V. C. *et al.* Effects of selective serotonin reuptake inhibitors on glaucoma: A nationwide population-based study. *PLoS One* 2017; **12**: e0173005, doi:10.1371/journal.pone.0173005.

14. Wang, H. Y. *et al.* The risk of glaucoma and serotonergic antidepressants: A systematic review and meta-analysis. *J Affect Disord* 2018; **241**: 63–70, doi:10.1016/j.jad.2018.07.079.

15. Zheng, W. *et al.* Systemic medication associations with presumed advanced or uncontrolled primary open-angle glaucoma. *Ophthalmology* 2018; **125**: 984–993, doi:10.1016/j.ophtha.2018.01.007.

16. Costagliola, C., *et al.* SSRIs and intraocular pressure modifications: evidence, therapeutic implications and possible mechanisms. *CNS Drugs* 2004; **18**: 475–484, doi:10.2165/00023210-200418080-00001.

17. Razeghinejad, M. R., Pro, M. J. & Katz, L. J. Non-steroidal drug-induced glaucoma. *Eye (Lond)* 2011; **25**: 971–980, doi:10.1038/eye.2011.128.

18. Jain, N. S., Ruan, C. W., Dhanji, S. R. & Symes, R. J. Psychotropic drug-induced glaucoma: A practical guide to diagnosis and management. *CNS Drugs* 2021; **35**: 283–289, doi:10.1007/s40263-020-00790-w.

19. Masís, M., Kakigi, C., Singh, K. & Lin, S. Association between self-reported bupropion use and glaucoma: a population-based study. *Br J Ophthalmol* 2017; **101**: 525–529, doi:10.1136/bjophthalmol-2016-308846.

20. Kahraman, N., Durmaz, O. & Durna, M. M. Mirtazapine-induced acute angle closure. *Indian J Ophthalmol* 2015; **63**: 539–540, doi:10.4103/0301-4738.162612.

21. Crooke, A., Colligris, B. & Pintor, J. Update in glaucoma medicinal chemistry: emerging evidence for the importance of melatonin analogues. *Curr Med Chem* 2012; **19**: 3508–3522, doi:10.2174/092986712801323234.

22. Pescosolido, N., Gatto, V., Stefanucci, A. & Rusciano, D. Oral treatment with the melatonin agonist agomelatine lowers the intraocular pressure of glaucoma patients. *Ophthalmic Physiol Opt* 2015; **35**: 201–205, doi:10.1111/opo.12189.

23. Agorastos, A. & Huber, C. G. The role of melatonin in glaucoma: implications concerning pathophysiological relevance and therapeutic potential. *J Pineal Res* 2011; **50**: 1–7, doi:10.1111/j.1600-079X.2010.00816.x.

24. Mahmut Onur Karaytug, M. E. D., Lut Tamam. Acute angle closure glaucoma induced by selective serotonin reuptake inhibitor, and reversed by agomelatine. *Cukurova Medical Journal* 2019; **44**: 1520–1523, doi:https://doi.org/10.17826/cumj.572186.

25. Souza, V. B. *et al.* Intraocular pressure in schizophrenic patients treated with psychiatric medications. *Arq Bras Oftalmol* 2008; **71**, 660–664, doi:10.1590/s0004-27492008000500009.

26. Achiron, A., Aviv, U., Mendel, L. & Burgansky-Eliash, Z. Acute angle closure glaucoma precipitated by olanzapine. *Int J Geriatr Psychiatry* 2015; **30**: 1101–1102, doi:10.1002/gps.4327.

27. Alarfaj, M. A. & Almater, A. I. Olanzapine-Induced acute angle closure. *Am J Case Rep* 2021; **22**: e934432, doi:10.12659/ajcr.934432.

28. Gökgöz Özişik, G. & Çağlar, Ç. Acute angle closure in a patient using olanzapine. *Psychiatr Danub* 2022; **34**: 306–307, doi:10.24869/psyd.2022.306.

29. Shen, E., Farukhi, S., Schmutz, M. & Mosaed, S. Acute angle-closure glaucoma associated with aripiprazole in the setting of plateau iris configuration. *J Glaucoma* 2018; **27**: e40–e43, doi:10.1097/ijg.0000000000000836.

30. Kimura, A. *et al.* Targeting oxidative stress for treatment of glaucoma and optic neuritis. *Oxid Med Cell Longev* 2017: 2817252, doi:10.1155/2017/2817252.

31. Kimura, A. *et al.* Valproic acid prevents retinal degeneration in a murine model of normal tension glaucoma. *Neurosci Lett* 2015; **588**: 108–113, doi:10.1016/j.neulet.2014.12.054.

32. Mahalingam, K. *et al.* Therapeutic potential of valproic acid in advanced glaucoma: A pilot study. *Indian J Ophthalmol* 2018; **66**: 1104–1108, doi:10.4103/ijo.IJO_108_18.

33. Singh, A., Kumar, T., Velagala, V. R., Thakre, S. & Joshi, A. The actions of lithium on glaucoma and other senile neurodegenerative diseases through GSK-3 inhibition: a narrative review. *Cureus* 2022; **14**: e28265, doi:10.7759/cureus.28265.

34. Vallée, A., Vallée, J. N. & Lecarpentier, Y. Lithium and atypical antipsychotics: the possible WNT/β pathway target in glaucoma. *Biomedicines* 2021; **9**: doi:10.3390/biomedicines9050473.

35. Huang, X., Wu, D. Y., Chen, G., Manji, H. & Chen, D. F. Support of retinal ganglion cell survival and axon regeneration by lithium through a Bcl-2-dependent mechanism. *Invest Ophthalmol Vis Sci* 2003; **44**: 347–354, doi:10.1167/iovs.02-0198.

36. Ah-Kee, E. Y., Egong, E., Shafi, A., Lim, L. T. & Yim, J. L. A review of drug-induced acute angle closure glaucoma for non-ophthalmologists. *Qatar Med J* 2015; **6**: doi:10.5339/qmj.2015.6.

37. Hu, W., Chen, L., Li, H. & Liu, J. Eye disorders associated with newer antiepileptic drugs: A real-world disproportionality analysis of FDA adverse event reporting system. *Seizure* 2022; **96**: 66–73, doi:10.1016/j.seizure.2022.01.011.

38. Ho, J.-D. *et al*. Topiramate Use and the risk of glaucoma development: a population-based follow-up study. *Am J Ophthalmology* 2013; **155**: 336–341.e331, doi: https://doi.org/10.1016/j.ajo.2012.07.016.

39. Etminan, M., Maberley, D. & Mikelberg, F. S. Use of topiramate and risk of glaucoma: a case-control study. *Am J Ophthalmology* 2012; **153**: 827–830.

Chapter 12

Starting Psychiatric Medicines after Overdose

CONTENTS

This chapter does not provide guidance on the acute management of drug toxicity from overdose. Refer to Toxbase or similar reference sources.

GENERAL PRINCIPLES

There are several factors to consider when deliberating about starting, or restarting, a psychiatric medication after an overdose of that drug. The most obvious concern is of safety: at what point can the patient be considered to have sufficiently 'cleared' the drug taken in overdose such that it is safe to either restart the drug, or commence an alternative psychiatric medication?

The Maudsley® Prescribing Guidelines for Mental Health Conditions in Physical Illness, First Edition.
Siobhan Gee and David M. Taylor.
© 2025 John Wiley & Sons Ltd. Published 2025 by John Wiley & Sons Ltd.

Before restarting a medication that has been taken in overdose, consideration should be given as to whether resuming the same drug is clinically appropriate and whether the medicine is still required. An overdose should be a prompt to review the effectiveness of the treatment being prescribed.

How quickly will the overdosed drug be eliminated from the body?

The elimination of most drugs follows first-order kinetics. The rate of removal is proportional to the plasma concentration of the drug and is best expressed by the drug's half-life, the time taken for the plasma concentration to halve.

It is often said that a drug can be considered completely removed from the body after five half-lives[1]. After one half-life, 50% of the initial total drug dose remains, after two half-lives 25% remains, after three half-lives 12.5%, after four half-lives 6.25%, and after five half-lives 3.125%. Whilst this rule may be useful in estimating a minimum time gap before recommencing treatment, it is by no means foolproof. For example, these percentages apply to the dose taken in overdose, which may be very large and give very high plasma concentrations (making even 3.125% of this blood level suprathera-peutic). If the overdose is sufficiently large, hepatic cytochrome P450 (CYP) enzyme function may become saturated, switching elimination to a zero-order model and delaying clearance still further.

Knowing the half-life of a particular drug does not provide certainty about its rate of elimination. Drug half-lives quoted in the literature, or by manufacturers, will inevitably describe an average. This is calculated from either single-dose or short-course pharmacokinetic studies, run in healthy volunteers, who are usually male and Caucasian. The actual half-life of a drug in an individual may be significantly different, influenced by many factors including other medication or substances that have been taken, and variations in CYP enzyme function. Even if all these patient-specific factors were taken into account, the half-life of a drug in overdose may be longer than in therapeutic use.

Other factors may also be important, depending on the drug in question. The absorption of the drug may be slowed if gastric transit time is increased (as for anticholinergic drugs), therefore slowing both the onset of toxicity and the eventual clearance of the overdose. The formulation taken may also be relevant, with sustained-release tablets or capsules slowing the rate of drug absorption and total elimination time. Sustained-release quetiapine tablets can form bezoars in the stomach, further slowing this process[2]. Drugs that rely wholly or in part on renal clearance (e.g. lithium) may have their clearance half-life extended if there is a decline in renal function – for example, if acute kidney injury accompanies the clinical presentation. Acute liver injury or reduction in hepatic blood flow may have the same effect for drugs metabolised in this way.

It is not only the parent drug but also the metabolites that must be considered – if pharmacologically active, the route of elimination for these must also be taken into account. For example, the didesmethyl metabolite of citalopram causes QT prolongation and seizures in high plasma concentrations. Check also for pharmacokinetic interactions with any other drugs taken before, during, or after the overdose. Drugs that inhibit CYP enzymes may slow the rate of metabolism of the drug taken in overdose, prolonging expected recovery times.

In some cases, elimination of drugs taken in overdose may be faster than expected, or plasma concentrations may be lower than expected in relation to the dose taken. If patients have vomited, some portion of the dose taken may not be absorbed. Smoking and other concurrent drugs can induce the metabolism of some psychiatric drugs (e.g. CYP metabolism of clozapine and olanzapine is induced by cigarette smoking). Drug elimination may also be increased depending on the treatment received for the overdose. For example, gut decontamination with activated charcoal can reduce the absorption of many drugs in patients presenting within one hour of a potentially toxic overdose, but its effectiveness decreases the longer the time gap is between overdose and administration.

ANTIDEPRESSANTS

Acute cardiovascular toxicity may present with refractory hypotension related to myocardial depression in tricyclic antidepressant (TCA) overdose. Acidosis, arrhythmias and seizures can exacerbate hypotension. ECGs typically demonstrate intraventricular conduction delay evident by QRS prolongation. The anticholinergic effect of TCAs may also prolong absorption times as gastric emptying is slowed[3]. Seizures and ECG changes, including prolongation of the QT interval predisposing to ventricular arrhythmias, may occur in SSRI overdoses (e.g. citalopram and escitalopram). Serotonin syndrome occurs most frequently following the use of combinations of serotonergic agents but may also occur following high therapeutic dosing or overdoses of a single drug (e.g. SSRIs, SNRIs).

Plasma concentrations of antidepressants are not routinely measured by most hospital pathology laboratories, and are unlikely to be readily available in a useful timeframe. Furthermore, for many drugs there is no established relationship between effect and serum concentration, making their interpretation problematic. When starting or restarting agents, the ECG (particularly QT and QRS intervals) and other cardiac parameters such as heart rate and blood pressure should be normal. Clinical signs and symptoms related to the overdose and related toxidromes may include dilated pupils, nystagmus, dizziness, ataxia, delirium, myoclonus, or muscle twitching. Patients may be observed to be picking at clothing or bedding due to ongoing anticholinergic effects. These signs should also be resolved before restarting.

ANTIPSYCHOTICS

Overdose with antipsychotics produces a range of symptoms affecting the central nervous and cardiovascular systems. Sedation is common, arising from histamine H_1 receptor blockade in the central nervous system, and is particularly pronounced with clozapine and quetiapine[4]. Profound CNS depression can lead to respiratory depression, and seizures are possible. Extrapyramidal syndromes may occur, including neuroleptic malignant syndrome, acute dystonia, and acute akathisia[5]. Cardiovascular toxicity may include hypotension, due to alpha-1 adrenergic mediated vasodilatation or impaired myocardial contractility[6]. Arrhythmias result from cardiac potassium channel blockade, causing prolongation of the QTc interval and torsades de pointes. Central and peripheral anticholinergic antagonism may cause hyperthermia, tachycardia, urinary retention, slowed bowel motility, and repetitive picking behaviour.

As for the antidepressants, plasma concentration monitoring is unlikely to be readily available (with the exception of clozapine, see below), and similarly does not always correlate well with clinical signs and symptoms. Check that the ECG and other cardiovascular parameters are normal before starting drugs after an antipsychotic overdose.

PRACTICAL ADVICE

Drug plasma concentrations have limited utility in the immediate evaluation and management of the acute overdose. Psychiatric medicines tend to have prolonged absorption phases and a wide variability in terminal elimination. Plasma concentrations may be used to guide a decision about whether and when to (re)start psychiatric medication, but they are often not routinely available, or not available in a meaningful timeframe. If they are quickly available, consider waiting until the plasma concentration reaches a therapeutic level (see table below) before starting psychiatric medication. Plasma concentration determinations may also be used to avoid inadvertently leaving a patient with subtherapeutic plasma concentrations (i.e. allowing restarting of medication before the plasma concentration drops to zero), and in the case of clozapine, avoiding the need for lengthy re-titration of doses.

In the majority of cases where plasma concentrations are not easily or usefully available, decisions about (re)starting medicines are based on a pragmatic approach, utilising pharmacological principles in the context of clinical signs and symptoms. The first step should always be to look at the patient. Does the patient appear toxic? Drowsy? Consider what adverse effects would be expected of the drug in question if the plasma concentration was high. For many drugs used in mental health this is sedation, but consider extrapyramidal side effects (antipsychotics), QT prolongation, and other ECG changes (antipsychotics and antidepressants). The physical health of the patient is more important than drug plasma concentrations.

Consider whether there are any adverse effects that would be particularly concerning for the patient, taking into account comorbidity and other medication. For example, a patient with a history of cardiac arrhythmia may be at heightened risk of antidepressant-induced arrhythmia. Patients with a history of epilepsy may have increased vulnerability to a reduction in seizure threshold from antipsychotic toxicity. Where adverse effects can be monitored, do so (e.g. ECG).

The risk of not prescribing needs to be balanced against the risk of adverse effects. In some cases, the drug taken in overdose was not effective for treatment of psychiatric symptoms, and patients can then continue to be mentally unwell despite having high plasma concentrations of psychiatric medication. If treatment cannot wait, then it may be necessary to administer sedatives such as benzodiazepines as an interim measure if it is unsafe to start another antipsychotic, antidepressant, or mood stabiliser. Consider the risks of starting a new drug before the one taken in overdose has been eliminated in the same way as if cross-tapering the medicines (antidepressant switching guidelines may be a useful tool to indicate potential risks, for example).

Clozapine

It is essential that plasma concentrations are used to guide reintroduction of clozapine after an overdose (of clozapine) has been taken. It is a drug with potential to be particularly toxic in overdose compared with other antipsychotics, and the plasma concentration may not decline in a predictably linear fashion (making the 'five half-lives' rule redundant). Case reports describe biphasic absorption of clozapine in overdose[7,8], and plateaus in plasma concentration lasting for several days. This may be a result of the slowed gastric emptying caused by the anticholinergic effects of clozapine, or CYP enzyme saturation. Concurrent inflammatory disease, including infection (pneumonia is common[9]), may impair metabolism and elimination[10].

The patient should be observed for cardiac adverse effects, notably hypotension, tachycardia, and QT prolongation and the associated risk of ventricular arrhythmia. Seizures are more likely at high plasma concentrations. CNS effects leading to reduced consciousness, coma, and respiratory depression may result in pneumonia due to aspiration of excessive hypersalivation. Acute renal failure has been reported[11], probably a consequence of reduced renal blood flow arising from hypotension.

If access to rapid turnaround plasma concentration testing is available (i.e. point-of-care testing), then it may be possible to restart clozapine before the plasma concentration drops to zero. If clozapine can be restarted when the plasma concentration is within the therapeutic range, then the usual slow dose titration can be avoided. The following guidance is suggested.

Plasma concentration (ng/ml)	Action
>500	Do not administer clozapine. Repeat plasma concentration in 24h.
100–500	Day 1: Give 50% of the usual maintenance dose in two divided doses. Day 2: Give the usual maintenance dose in two divided doses.
>0 but <100	Day 1: Give 25% of the usual maintenance dose in two divided doses. Day 2: Give 50% of the usual maintenance dose in two divided doses. Day 3: Give the usual maintenance dose in two divided doses.

Note that dose increases should only be given if the previous dose was tolerated – if tachycardia, hypotension, or drowsiness occurs, then revert to the previously tolerated dose (or withhold clozapine for a further 12–24h before attempting to restart again).

Summary

- Following overdose, observe the patient for signs of adverse effects / toxicity (refer to Toxbase for the management of acute toxicity).
- If plasma concentrations are available, they may be used to determine when a level reaches the therapeutic range, but note that many drugs do not have a well-established relationship between effect and serum concentration.

CHAPTER 12

- If the plasma concentration is not available, use the total amount of drug taken and the half-life to calculate the time at which the plasma concentration is likely to be within therapeutic range. If the drug taken has active metabolites, use the longest half-life of the active moieties.
- If plasma concentrations are not available and the amount of drug taken is unknown, calculate five half-lives and use this as a guide amount of time to wait before starting or restarting a psychiatric medication. If the drug taken has active metabolites, use the longest half-life of the active moiety.
- Overdose histories are frequently not disclosed, or are unreliable. If there are minimal clinical signs and symptoms, it may not be justifiable to withhold treatments for periods as long as indicated by calculations based on half-lives. In these cases, take a pragmatic approach and consider restarting medicines after 1–2 days.
- Only restart a drug (or start a new drug) if the patient is medically fit to do so (i.e. showing no signs of toxicity, observations are normal, ECG is normal). Avoid starting more than one drug at a time.
- Ideally, observe the patient (in hospital or at home) for at least 3–5 days after a drug is (re)started. If this is not possible, advise patients to seek medical advice if they feel unwell after discharge.
- In all cases, use clinical judgement – do not start medicines if the patient is unwell and it is unsafe to do so. Conversely, it may be possible to start medicines earlier than outlined above if the patient is physically well and there is a clinical need to do so.

Worked examples

For a patient who has taken 300mg of olanzapine, plasma concentration is unknown. The half-life of olanzapine may be up to 60h; therefore:

- After 60h the effective dose is 150mg.
- After 120h = 75mg.
- After 180h = 37.5mg.
- After 240h = 18.75mg – within normal dose range; the patient could start at 20mg.
- After 300h = 9.375mg – within normal dose range; the patient could start at 10mg.

For a patient who has taken 600mg of venlafaxine, plasma concentration is unknown. The half-life of venlafaxine is up to 14h, with an active metabolite half-life of up to 20h; therefore:

- After 20h the effective dose is 300mg.
- After 40h the effective dose is 150mg – within normal range, the patient could restart.

THERAPEUTIC REFERENCE RANGES AND HALF-LIVES

Drug (active metabolite)	Therapeutic reference range (ng/ml)[12]	Half-life (active metabolite)[12]	Specific considerations[13]
		Antidepressants	
TCAs			Prolonged QRS/ QT, cardiac arrhythmia, hypotension, anticholinergic effects, seizures
Amitriptyline (nortriptyline)	80–200	Amitriptyline 10–28h (18–44h)	
Clomipramine (N-desmethylclomipramine)	230–450	Clomipramine 16–60h (37–43h)	
Dosulepin	45–100	18–21h	
Imipramine (desipramine)	175–300	11–25h (15–18h)	
Nortriptyline	70–170	18–44h	
Trimipramine	150–300	23–24h	
SSRIs and SNRIs			Serotonin syndrome
Fluvoxamine	60–230	21–43h	Seizures
Sertraline	10–150	22–36h	
Paroxetine	20–65	12–44h	
Citalopram	50–110	38–48h	Prolonged QT
Escitalopram	15–80	27–32h	Prolonged QT
Fluoxetine (N-desmethylfluoxetine)	120–500	4–6 days (4–15 days)	
Venlafaxine XL (O-desmethylvenlafaxine)	100–400	4–14h (10–20h)	Prolonged QT, hypertension, tachycardia, seizures
Duloxetine	30–120	9–19h	Seizures
Vortioxetine	10–40	57–66h	
MAOIs			Tachycardia, seizures
Moclobemide	300–1000	2–7h	Hyperreflexia, serotonin syndrome
Tranylcypromine	< 50	1–3h	Hyperthermia, hypertension
Others			
Agomelatine	7–300	1–2h	
Bupropion (+ hydroxybupropion)	850–1500	1–15h (17–47h)	
Mianserin	15–70	13–33h	
Mirtazapine	30–80	20–40h	Sedation, hypotension, tachycardia
Trazodone	700–1000	4–11h	

(Continued)

CHAPTER 12

Drug (active metabolite)	Therapeutic reference range (ng/ml)[12]	Half-life (active metabolite)[12]	Specific considerations[13]
		Antipsychotics	
Typicals			EPSEs, QT prolongation, sedation
Chlorpromazine	30–300	15–30h	Seizures
Flupenthixol	0.5–5	20–40h	
Haloperidol	1–10	12–36h	
Pimozide	15–20	23–43h	
Sulpiride	200–1000	8–14h	
Zuclopenthixol	4–50	15–25h	
Atypicals			QT prolongation, sedation
Amisulpride	100–230	12–20h	Renally cleared
Quetiapine (N-desalkylquetiapine)	100–500	6–11h (10–13h)	Seizures, tachycardia
Aripiprazole (dehydroaripiprazole)	100–350	60–80h (30–47h)	Orthostatic hypotension, tachycardia
Asenapine	1–5	13–39h	
Cariprazine	10–20	48–120h	
Clozapine	350–500	12–16h	Tachycardia, seizures, hypersalivation
Lurasidone	15–40	20–40h	
Olanzapine	20–80	30–60h	Arrhythmias
Paliperidone	20–60	17–23h	
Risperidone (paliperidone)	20–60	2–4h (17–23h)	Tachycardia, heart block
Mood stabilisers			
Carbamazepine	4–10mcg/ml	10–20h	
Lamotrigine	1–6mcg/ml	14–104h	
Lithium	0.5–1.2mmol/l	14–30h	
Sodium valproate	50–100mcg/ml	11–17h	

References

1. Andrade, C. The practical importance of half-life in psychopharmacology. *J Clin Psychiatry* 2022; **83**, doi:10.4088/JCP.22f14584.

2. Rauber-Lüthy, C. et al. Gastric pharmacobezoars in quetiapine extended-release overdose: a case series. *Clin Toxicol (Phila)* 2013; **51**: 937–940, doi:10.3109/15563650.2013.856442.

3. Adams, B. K., Mann, M. D., Aboo, A., Isaacs, S. & Evans, A. Prolonged gastric emptying half-time and gastric hypomotility after drug overdose. *Am J Emerg Med* 2004; **22**: 548–554, doi:10.1016/j.ajem.2004.08.017.

4. Minns, A. B. & Clark, R. F. Toxicology and overdose of atypical antipsychotics. *J Emerg Med* 2012; **43**: 906–913, doi:10.1016/j.jememed.2012.03.002.

5. Levine, M. & Ruha, A.-M. Overdose of Atypical Antipsychotics. *CNS Drugs* 2012; **26**: 601–611, doi:10.2165/11631640-000000000-00000.

6. Tan, H. H., Hoppe, J. & Heard, K. A systematic review of cardiovascular effects after atypical antipsychotic medication overdose. *Am J Emerg Med* 2009; **27**: 607–616, doi:10.1016/j.ajem.2008.04.020.

7. Thomas, L. & Pollak, P. T. Delayed recovery associated with persistent serum concentrations after clozapine overdose. *J Emerg Med* 2003; **25**: 61–66, doi:10.1016/s0736-4679(03)00130-6.

8. Hägg, S., Spigset, O., Edwardsson, H. & Björk, H. Prolonged sedation and slowly decreasing clozapine serum concentrations after an overdose. *J Clin Psychopharmacol* 1999; **19**: 282–284, doi:10.1097/00004714-199906000-00019.

9. Mace, S. et al. Incident infection during the first year of treatment – A comparison of clozapine and paliperidone palmitate long-acting injection. *J Psychopharmacol* 2022; **36**: 232–237, doi:10.1177/02698811211058973.

10. Davis, E. A. K., Hightower, T. & Cinnamon, K. A. Toxic clozapine level as first indication of severe, acute infection. *Ment Health Clin* 2022; **12**, 45–48, doi:10.9740/mhc.2022.01.045.

11. Daaboul, A., Sedding, D., Nuding, S. & Schott, A. Successful treatment of an acute high-dose clozapine poisoning without detoxication. *Am J Case Rep* 2021; **22**: e929147. doi:10.12659/ajcr.929147.

12. Hiemke, C. et al. Consensus Guidelines for Therapeutic Drug Monitoring in Neuropsychopharmacology: Update 2017. *Pharmacopsychiatry* 2018; **51**: 9–62.

13. Tay, E. et al. Restarting antidepressant and antipsychotic medication after intentional overdoses: need for evidence-based guidance. *Ther Adv Psychopharmacol* 2019; **9**. doi:10.1177/2045125319836889.

CHAPTER 12

Chapter 13

Non-oral Routes of Administration

CONTENTS

The Maudsley® Prescribing Guidelines for Mental Health Conditions in Physical Illness, First Edition.
Siobhan Gee and David M. Taylor.
© 2025 John Wiley & Sons Ltd. Published 2025 by John Wiley & Sons Ltd.

Oral administration of medicines may not always be possible. Patients may be unable or unwilling to take medicines orally, or gastrointestinal absorption of medication may be compromised. Alternative treatments such as psychological interventions and electroconvulsive therapy (ECT) are often either impractical or contra-indicated in the medically unwell patient. In these circumstances, clinicians may look to administer medicines by other routes.

In some scenarios, it may be necessary to consider indications and routes of administration that are outside standard labelling. For example, psychotropics that are not conventionally labelled antidepressants may possess pharmacological antidepressant activity, and may be more readily available in non-oral formulations. Many of the atypical antipsychotics are available as intramuscular injections, although data supporting use in depression are limited to oral adjunct of standard antidepressants. But when faced with few to zero alternative treatment options, a trial of a drug with the desired pharmacological properties, even if not the relevant licensed indication, may be worthwhile.

Use of off-label formulations or licensed formulations via unlicensed routes (crushing tablets, administering via enteral feeding tubes) requires documentation of the reasoning for the choice of treatment and route, as with all unlicensed preparations[1]. If at all possible, every effort should be made to outline this reasoning to the patient and/or their next of kin. Prescribers should note the restrictions and guidelines associated with product licensing relevant to their country of practice.

ENTERAL FEEDING TUBES

If the patient has a feeding tube in place, medicines can usually be administered using this route. Enteral feeding tubes can be inserted via the nasopharynx into the stomach (nasogastric, NG) or jejunum (nasojejunal, NJ). Alternately, the tube may be inserted directly into the gastrointestinal tract through the skin, either into the stomach (percutaneous endoscopic gastrostomy, PEG) or jejunum (jejunostomy, often a PEG with an extension into the jejunum, PEG-J). Wide-bore tubes may be inserted NG and used for aspiration or drainage (Ryles tubes). Ryles tubes cannot usually be used for medicine administration unless it is possible to temporarily pause the drainage. (It is worth checking whether this is the case.)

Delivery of drugs via NG or PEG would be expected to afford little change in pharmacokinetics, since most drug absorption occurs in the small intestine, distal to the point of delivery via the tube. However, scant data are published describing either plasma concentrations or patient outcomes when psychotropics are delivered via enteral tubes. One case report found reduced plasma concentrations of clozapine using a PEG[2]. Delivery of drugs via gastric access devices can be influenced by enteral feeds, resulting in reduced absorption (e.g. tetracyclines, levothyroxine, bisphosphonates), premature degradation and activation (proton pump inhibitors), increased absorption (carbamazepine), or chelation (warfarin, tetracyclines, phenytoin)[3].

Administration into the jejunum ('postpyloric', NJ or PEG-J) may be more problematic for drug delivery than NG routes. Both increased and decreased absorption can occur. Increased absorption may result because of the reduced opportunity for degradation by stomach acid or reduced first-pass metabolism[4]. Reduced absorption may be a consequence of the missed opportunity for absorption in the duodenum.

The position of the tube may also cause problems, as the distal point of the tube can migrate along the gastrointestinal tract, potentially delivering medication to sites other than those considered optimal for absorption[3]. Tube occlusion can occur; it is more likely if drugs are inadequately suspended (e.g. with large insoluble solid particles) and if the tubes are narrow and/or longer[3].

Reliable information on exactly where in the gastrointestinal tract various drugs are absorbed is lacking. In most scenarios, this information is redundant in respect to choice since alternative options for administration may be very limited, if available at all. In general, if an enteral tube can be used for medicines administration it is better to try this route and observe response rather than dismissing it for fear of lack of drug absorption.

Where possible, use commercial liquid formulations of drugs to administer via enteral tubes. These will either be solutions or suspensions of non-clumping fine particles. Orodispersible formulations can be dispersed in water. If no liquid formulation is available, in the majority of cases there is little risk to crushing tablets. The absence of evidence for doing this should not be a barrier if there is nothing about the formulation of the tablet that obviously precludes crushing. Crushing should aim to reduce particle size to a minimum.

The use of plasma concentrations to guide dosing when using enteral feeding tubes is recommended when using drugs with a narrow therapeutic index (clozapine, lithium). Plasma level monitoring may also be helpful for some cases in differentiating between non-response and lack of absorption.

ANTIDEPRESSANTS

Very few non-oral formulations of antidepressants are available as commercial products. Most formulations do not have formal licences and may be very difficult to obtain, being available only through pharmaceutical importers or from Specials manufacturers.

Sublingual

There are a small number of case reports supporting the effectiveness of **fluoxetine** liquid used sublingually in depressed, medically compromised patients[5]. In these reports, doses of up to 60mg a day produced plasma fluoxetine and norfluoxetine levels towards the lower end of the proposed therapeutic range[5]. **Ketamine** injection has also been used sublingually, with apparent good efficacy[6]. It may be better tolerated than other routes of administration (IV or SC)[6].

Buccal

Selegiline is available as oral lyophilisates for absorption in the buccal cavity (licensed for the treatment of Parkinson's disease), but is selective for MAO-B inhibition at the 1.25mg doses available. A lack of action at MAO-A in the central nervous system at these doses is thought to preclude antidepressant activity[7]. A very small study of orally disintegrating 10mg/day selegiline, however, showed significant inhibition of brain MAO-A, but clinical antidepressant activity has not been investigated[8].

CHAPTER 13

One case report describes buccal administration of **amitriptyline** tablets[9] achieving therapeutic plasma levels. Another case used orodispersible **mirtazapine** assuming buccal absorption[10], although no plasma levels were reported. No information is available to suggest that orodispersible mirtazapine is actually absorbed through the buccal mucosa (as opposed to dispersing in saliva that is then swallowed).

Intravenous and intramuscular

Intravenous formulations of antidepressants avoid the first pass effect, leading to somewhat higher drug plasma levels[11,12] and perhaps greater response[12,13], but not necessarily faster onset of action[13-16]. The placebo effect associated with IV administration is known to be large[17]. Calculating the correct parenteral dose of antidepressants is difficult given the variable first pass effect to which oral drugs are usually subject. Parenteral doses can be expected to be much lower than oral doses and give the same effect.

Intravenous **citalopram** followed by maintenance oral citalopram may be a clinically useful treatment strategy for severely depressed, hospitalised patients[14]. Better efficacy and faster response (compared with oral doses) have also been demonstrated when using IV citalopram in treating symptoms of obsessive compulsive disorder[18]. The IV preparation appears to be well-tolerated; the most common adverse events are nausea, headache, tremor, and somnolence, similar to oral administration[19,20]. A case report of a 65-year-old man described acute hyperkinetic delirium associated with IV citalopram[21]. Intravenous **escitalopram** is described in the literature, although studies reported to date are pharmacokinetic analyses[22]. Oral citalopram is associated with a higher risk of QTc prolongation than other SSRIs. If used IV in a medically compromised patient, ECG monitoring is recommended.

Mirtazapine has been administered by slow infusion at a dose of 15mg/day for 14 days in two studies and was well tolerated[23,24]. There are reports of IV mirtazapine 6–30mg/day being used to treat hyperemesis gravidarum[25,26], but the intravenous preparation does not appear to be commercially available.

Amitriptyline was available as both an IV and IM injection (IM injection has been given IV) and both routes have been used in the treatment of postoperative pain and depression[27]. The concentration of the IM preparation (10mg/ml) may mean a high volume injection is needed to achieve antidepressant doses and this clearly militates against its use intramuscularly[28]. It is no longer available in most parts of the world.

Clomipramine is probably the most widely studied IV antidepressant. Pulse-loading doses of intravenous clomipramine have been shown to produce a larger and more rapid decrease in obsessive compulsive disorder symptoms compared with oral doses[11,29]. The potential for serious cardiac side effects when using any tricyclic antidepressant intravenously necessitates monitoring of pulse, blood pressure and ECG.

Injectable **trazodone** is available in Italy for intramuscular or intravenous use. Small studies demonstrate efficacy in depression[30], and psychomotor agitation in bipolar disorder[31,32]. Sedation is common.

Allopregnanolone (marketed as **brexanolone**) is an endogenous progesterone metabolite licensed in the USA for intravenous treatment of postpartum depression. Given the unique mechanism of action, it is probably not suitable for treatment of other types of depression.

Extensive studies of IV **ketamine**, a glutamate N-methyl-d-aspartate (NMDA) receptor antagonist, have demonstrated rapid, albeit short-lived antidepressant effects[33]. Concerns over long-term duration of response may be less relevant for acutely medically unwell patients. Ketamine has also been delivered via intranasal[34], IM, and SC routes[35,36], sublingually[6,37] and via transmucosal routes[38].

IV and IM **scopolamine (hyoscine)** as an antidepressant has also been investigated. Studies to date have been conflicting, with some failing to demonstrate any effect in depression and others suggesting rapid antidepressant effects within 72h in both unipolar and bipolar depression[39-42]. Anticholinergic adverse effects are likely (blurred vision, dry mouth, drowsiness, dizziness, tachycardia, anxiety).

Flupentixol long-acting intramuscular injection has been used in low doses for the treatment of depression[43].

Transdermal

Amitriptyline gel is used in pain clinics as an adjuvant in the treatment of a variety of chronic pain conditions[44,45]. It is usually prepared as a 50mmol/L or 100mmol/L gel with or without lidocaine. Although it has proven analgesic activity, there are no published data on the plasma levels attained via this route. **Nortriptyline** hydrochloride has been formulated as a transdermal patch for smoking cessation[46]. Nanoemulsion formulations of **imipramine** and of **doxepin** have also been formulated for transdermal delivery for use as analgesics[47]. At the time of writing, there are no published studies on nortriptyline patches or imipramine or doxepin nanoemulsions in depression. It is unlikely that any of these formulations achieve plasma concentrations high enough to elicit antidepressant effects.

Oral **selegiline** at doses greater than 20mg/day may be antidepressant, but enzyme selectivity is lost at these doses, necessitating a tyramine-restricted diet[48,49]. Selegiline can instead be administered transdermally[50]. Selegiline patches, marketed as Emsam™, deliver 25–30% of the selegiline content over 24h; steady-state plasma concentrations are achieved within 5 days of daily dosing[51]. This route bypasses first-pass metabolism, thereby providing a higher, more sustained, plasma concentration of selegiline while being relatively sparing of the gastrointestinal MAO-A system[52,53]. There seems to be no need for tyramine restriction when the lower dose patch (6mg/24h) is used, and there have been no reports of hypertensive reactions even with the higher-dose patch. Patients using the higher-strength patches (9 or 12mg/24h) should avoid very high tyramine content food substances[54] but generally transdermal selegiline is well tolerated.

Rectal

The rectal mucosa lacks the extensive villi and microvilli of other parts of the gastrointestinal tract, limiting its surface area. Therefore rectal agents need to be in a formulation that maximises the extent of contact the active ingredient will have with the mucosa. There are no readily available antidepressant suppositories, but extemporaneous preparation is possible. For example, **amitriptyline** (in cocoa butter) suppositories have been manufactured by a hospital pharmacy and administered in a dose of 50mg twice daily with some subjective success[55,56]. **Doxepin** capsules have been administered via the rectal route directly in the treatment of cancer-related pain (without a special formulation) and produced plasma concentrations within the supposed therapeutic range[57]. Similarly, it has been reported that extemporaneously manufactured **imipramine** and **clomipramine** suppositories produced plasma levels comparable with the oral route of administration[58]. **Trazodone** has also been successfully administered in a suppository formulation postoperatively for a patient who was stable on the oral formulation prior to surgery[56,57]. **Sertraline** tablets administered rectally have also been used with success in a critically ill patient with bowel compromise[59].

Intranasal

Esketamine is available as a nasal spray (Spravato) and was licensed in the UK in 2019 and in the USA in 2020 for treatment-resistant major depressive disorder. It requires specific administration practices (tilting of the head, sniffing), which may not be possible to adhere to in medically unwell patients. At the time of writing, the UK National Institute of Health and Care Excellence had not recommended intranasal esketamine for use in treatment-resistant depression due to concerns over clinical- and cost-effectiveness (in long-term use). This may make it difficult to obtain in UK hospitals, where ketamine (in other formulations) is cheap and readily available.

ANTIPSYCHOTICS

Sublingual

Asenapine is manufactured as a sublingual tablet. Once placed under the tongue, the tablet dissolves in saliva within seconds, and peak plasma concentrations are attained within 0.5–1.5h[60]. The bioavailability of asenapine is very low if the tablet is swallowed (less than 2%).

The orodispersible formulation of **olanzapine** is not designed for sublingual use. As for other orodispersible preparations, the tablets dissolve in saliva, which is then swallowed. Drug absorption occurs in the gastrointestinal tract, not buccally. This limits the usefulness of orodispersible preparations for patients who lack a functioning gastrointestinal tract. However, two case reports describe successful 'sublingual' use of orodispersible olanzapine in end of life care[61,62]. One study in 10 healthy volunteers given sublingual orordispersible olanzapine demonstrated attainment of plasma concentrations comparable to standard oral tablets and normal use of the orodispersible formulation[63]. (In this study, participants held dispersible olanzapine in their mouths for 15min and 'were encouraged not to swallow'.)

Haloperidol ampoules have been used sublingually in end of life care for the management of agitation, nausea, and vomiting[64].

Intramuscular

Short-acting intramuscular preparations are commercially available for **haloperidol, droperidol, ziprasidone, chlorpromazine, fluphenazine, aripiprazole,** and **olanzapine. Zuclopenthixol acetate** (marketed as Acuphase) is given intramuscularly and is rapidly absorbed but slow to act. Sedation may occur within 2–4h, but antipsychotic action is evident after 8h[65].

When **clozapine** was first marketed in the 1990s, an IM formulation (50mg/2ml[66]) was available alongside the oral tablet, at least in Europe and Israel[66,67]. This was withdrawn in 2005 by the manufacturer (initially Sandoz, and later Novartis) for commercial reasons[68], and thereafter parenteral clozapine was only available from compounding pharmacies[69,70], severely curtailing accessibility. More recently, an IM product has been produced by Apotheek A15 (formally Brocacef), a Dutch manufacturer, and El Saad Pharma (based in Syria). Experience is growing with use, particularly in the UK[71-74] and the Netherlands[75].

The strength of the injection is 25mg/ml, with each ampoule containing 5ml (125mg). It is administered by deep IM injection and may be painful (a problem also noted with the original Sandoz product[67,76]). The formation of nodules at the injection site is reported, possibly linked to the length of treatment[72,73]. It is usually given into the gluteal muscle (and this is the route specified for the Dutch product), but the deltoid has also been used where the patient's body habitus prompted concerns that the gluteal would be difficult to access[71]. Due to the low oral bioavailability of clozapine and the assumption of 100% bioavailability for parenteral administration, usual practice is to halve the oral dose for IM dosing and to give the injection once daily (more frequent (twice daily) administration schedules have also been used[77]). It should be noted that to date, no pharmacokinetic studies have been published for the IM formulation. The maximum amount that is usually injected into any site is 4ml (100mg); doses greater than this must be split over different injection sites[72]. This clearly limits the potential for achieving therapeutic plasma concentrations in some patients (although some patients are reported to have received up to 500mg daily IM[70], but local abscesses are described with such high injected volumes[66]). In practice, the experience of most clinicians is for patients to either not require IM clozapine at all (the suggestion of this as a treatment plan is sufficient to encourage oral compliance), or require only a few doses before oral treatment is accepted[66,70,73].

The majority of authors describe the use of IM clozapine as an enforced treatment strategy, used where patients refuse to comply with oral therapy, but there is also a role for the formulation in cases where oral treatment is not possible for medical reasons[71]. Published case series describe a high degree of success with IM treatment, where success is considered to be achievement of compliance with oral clozapine, but also in achieving control of psychotic symptoms in cases where oral medicines administration is medically precluded[70,71]. Most patients receiving IM treatment due to refusal of oral clozapine are reported to require a week or less of injections[78] before conversion to oral therapy is possible, with high proportions (90–100% in some studies[66]) going on to accept oral clozapine.

CHAPTER 13

Long-acting intramuscular injections (depots) are commercially available for **haloperidol, flupenthixol, fluphenazine, pipothiazine, zuclopenthixol, aripiprazole, olanzapine, risperidone,** and **paliperidone.**

Intravenous

Haloperidol can be given intravenously, but continuously cardiac monitoring is recommended if this route is used (see Chapter 7, Delirium, for further discussion). **Droperidol** can also be given intravenously and is usually used for postoperative nausea and vomiting. A Cochrane review supports the use of droperidol for acute psychosis[79]. The onset of action is 3–10min, with a peak effect at 30min. Sedation may last 2–4h.

The short-acting intramuscular preparation of **olanzapine** can be given as an IV bolus. Peak plasma concentrations are considerably higher than with oral olanzapine, so as for IM administration, doses should be initially low (1.25–2.5mg) and increased if necessary to a maximum of 10mg as a single dose. If parenteral benzodiazepines are given concurrently to IV olanzapine, monitor for cardiorespiratory depression, a complication reported (albeit not consistently) with the combination of IM olanzapine and IM benzodiazepines[80].

Subcutaneous

Haloperidol is commonly delivered subcutaneously via syringe drivers in palliative care[81]. A once-monthly SC administered formulation of **risperidone** is licensed in the USA (Uzedy™)[82]. SC administration of **olanzapine** is described in the literature either for use in delirium[83], or managing psychosis at the end of life[84]. The short-acting IM formulation can be given SC as a bolus injection. A maximum single dose of 10mg is recommended due to higher peak plasma concentrations achieved using parenteral olanzapine compared with oral. Doses can be given twice[84], or even three times[83] daily if required. Continuous SC infusion over 24h using a syringe driver has also been described[84]. **Fluphenazine** long-acting injection is licensed in the USA to be given subcutaneously.

Transdermal

Blonanserin is available as a transdermal patch in Japan and Korea. **Asenapine** transdermal patches are marketed in the USA.

Inhalation

Loxapine is available in a single-dose, disposable inhalation device designed for the acute treatment of agitation in schizophrenia or bipolar disorder. It is rapidly absorbed, and peak plasma concentrations are achieved within 2min. There is a risk of bronchospasm, and inhaled loxapine is contraindicated for patients with a history of lung disease (including asthma and COPD).

MOOD STABILISERS

Intravenous

Sodium valproate is available as an IV injection that can be given directly or by infusion.

Subcutaneous

Sodium valproate can be given via SC infusion. SC doses described in the literature (for seizure control in palliative care) range from 500 to 2500mg/day[85].

Rectal

Carbamazepine suppositories are commercially available. **Lamotrigine** tablets[86] and dispersible tablets[87] have been used rectally in the management of seizures[88], although absorption is lower than for oral administration. **Topiramate** tablets have been crushed and dispersed in 10ml of water for rectal administration, with a small pharmacokinetic study demonstrating similar bioavailability to the oral route[89]. **Sodium valproate** liquid, diluted in a 1:1 ratio with tap water[90] has been administered rectally for seizures in children and adults[89]. **Oxcarbazepine** liquid was given rectally in a pharmacokinetic study, but plasma concentrations failed to reach therapeutic levels, probably because of poor water solubility[91].

OTHER DRUGS

A sublingual/buccal film of **dexmedetomidine** is marketed in some countries as a treatment for acute agitation associated with schizophrenia and bipolar disorder[92].

SUMMARY

Drug	Dosing Information	Manufacturer	Notes
Sublingual			
Fluoxetine	Doses up to 60mg/day	Use liquid fluoxetine preparation	Plasma levels are likely to be lower compared with oral dosing.
Ketamine	Regular lower doses: ■ 0.5–1.5mg/kg every 1–3 days ■ Limited evidence for very low SL dosing (10mg every 2–3 days or weekly) Intermittent higher doses to supplement IV/SC/IM doses: ■ 1.5–3mg/kg once or twice a week	Use ketamine solution held under the tongue for 5min, then swallowed, or use ketamine lozenges	Lower doses given SL are well tolerated but may not be as rapidly effective as other routes (IV, SC, IM).
Asenapine	5–10mg twice daily	Organon Pharma (UK)	Asenapine is the only psychotropic medicine that has been formulated specifically for SL absorption.

Drug	Dosing Information	Manufacturer	Notes
Olanzapine	10–20mg daily	Generic orodispersible preparation	Orodispersible preparations are not designed for SL absorption; plasma concentrations are likely to be lower compared with oral dosing.
Haloperidol	Low doses (0.25–0.5mg) used in end of life care	Use the parenteral ampoules or liquid preparation	Only described in management of nausea and vomiting in end of life care, where doses are very low.
Dexmedetomidine	Recommended doses depend on severity of agitation, degree of hepatic impairment, and age. See product literature.	BioXcel Therapeutics	Designed for sublingual or buccal administration. Patient must not eat or drink for 15min after sublingual administration, or 1h after buccal administration. Dose-dependent hypotension and bradycardia may occur.

Buccal			
Selegiline (oral lyophilisate)	10mg (8 × 1.25mg lyophilisates) daily	Cephalon UK Limited	Orally disintegrating freeze-dried formulation (Zelapar®) is licensed for treatment of Parkinson's disease. Trial data showed that 10mg of the lyophilizate formulation was required for MAO-A inhibition[8] – this may be practically difficult to administer.
Amitriptyline	Initiated at 25mg nocte and titrated up to 125mg/day	Generic amitriptyline	Tablets were crushed and allowed to dissolve in patient's mouth to promote buccal absorption. Authors report a decrease in the patient's depression[9].
Mirtazapine	15–45mg/day	Generic orodisperisble preparation	Orodispersible preparations are not designed for buccal absorption; plasma concentrations are likely to be lower compared with oral dosing.

Intravenous			
Amitriptyline	25–100mg given in 250ml sodium chloride intravenous infusion 0.9% by slow infusion over 120min	Contact local importer	Adverse effects tend to be dose-related and are largely similar to the oral formulation. At higher doses, drowsiness and dizziness occur. Bradycardia may occur with doses around 100mg. ECG monitoring is recommended.

Drug	Dosing Information	Manufacturer	Notes
Clomipramine	25mg/2ml injection Starting dose is 25mg diluted in 500ml sodium chloride intravenous infusion 0.9% given by slow infusion over 90min. Increased to 250–300mg in increments of 25mg/day over 10–14 days[93,94].	Novartis Defiante	The most common reported side effects are similar to the oral formulation, which included nausea, sweating, restlessness, flushing, drowsiness, fatigue, abdominal distress, and nervousness. ECG monitoring is recommended.
	Another report used starting dose of 50mg IV per day and titrated up to a maximum dose of 225mg/day over 5–7 days[95].		Reduction of symptoms was detected after 1 week of the first IV dose.
Citalopram	40mg/ml injection Doses from 20–40mg in 250ml sodium chloride intravenous infusion 0.9% or glucose 5%. Doses up to 80mg have been used for OCD. Rate of infusion is 20mg/h.	Lundbeck – available in some countries Can be imported from Germany but may take 3–4 weeks to obtain	The most commonly reported side effects are nausea, headache, tremor and somnolence, similar to adverse effects of the oral preparation. A case of acute hyperkinetic delirium has also been reported. Used for depression and obsessive compulsive disorder. ECG monitoring is recommended.
Escitalopram	10mg slow infusion over 60min	Lundbeck – not marketed anywhere in the world	Studies to date have only looked at pharmacokinetic profile. ECG monitoring is recommended.
Mirtazapine	6mg/2ml infusion solution 15mg/5ml infusion solution Dose 15mg in glucose 5% over 60min	Not marketed anywhere in the world	The most common reported side effects are nausea, sedation, and dizziness similar to side effects of the oral preparation.
Trazodone[30,31,96]	25–100mg in 250ml of sodium chloride intravenous infusion 0.9% daily for 1 week, lasting approximately 1.5h. IV doses were decided according to the severity of depressive symptoms.	Available only in Italy	Trazodone showed a significant improvement of symptoms after only 1 week of IV treatment and was better tolerated than clomipramine.
Brexanolone	Continuous infusion over 60h: ■ 0–4h: Initiate with a dosage of 30mcg/kg/h ■ 4–24h: Increase dosage to 60mcg/kg/h ■ 24–52h: Increase dosage to 90mcg/kg/h (alternatively consider a dosage of 60mcg/kg/h for those who do not tolerate 90mcg/kg/h) ■ 52–56h: Decrease dosage to 60mcg/kg/h ■ 56–60h: Decrease dosage to 30mcg/kg/h	Sage Therapeutics Inc.	Suitable only for postpartum depression

CHAPTER 13

Drug	Dosing Information	Manufacturer	Notes
Ketamine	Infusion over 40min: ■ 0.5mg/kg, increasing up to 1mg/kg if no response ■ Titrate from 0.25mg/kg in elderly patients	Generic ketamine	Cognitive effects (confusion, dissociation) occasionally occur Associated with transient increase in BP, tachycardia, and arrhythmias. Pretreatment ECG and pre/post BP monitoring are required.
Scopolamine	Infusion of 4mcg/kg every 3–4 days[97]	Generic scopolamine	Very limited evidence; not recommended Anticholinergic adverse effects are common: blurred vision, dry mouth, drowsiness, dizziness, tachycardia, anxiety Higher doses (6mcg/kg) failed to show antidepressant efficacy in one trial[98]
Haloperidol	Start at low dose (1–2mg) and titrate to response	Use the short-acting IM preparation.	IV use not approved by manufacturers Continuous ECG monitoring recommended, particularly for doses >5mg (dose-dependent risk of QT prolongation)[99]
Droperidol[79]	Slow IV bolus 5–15mg repeated every 4–6h	Generic droperidol	Pre-treatment ECG required
Olanzapine	IV bolus Initially 1.25–2.5mg; increase if necessary to a maximum of 10mg as a single dose	Use the short-acting IM preparation	Peak plasma concentrations are considerably higher with IM or IV dosing than oral. Avoid concurrent parenteral benzodiazepines if possible – risk of cardiorespiratory depression.
Sodium valproate[100]	20–30mg/kg as a slow IV injection over 3–5min, or continuous infusion, up to a maximum of 2500mg/day Oral doses can be converted directly into intravenous doses	Generic sodium valproate	Note that hypoalbuminaemia is common in medically unwell patients and will increase the free fraction of valproate. Dose cautiously in these circumstances. Monitor for hepatoxicity, pancreatitis, thrombocytopaenia, and hyperammonaemia in medically unwell patients.
Intramuscular			
Flupentixol decanoate depot[43]	5–10mg/2 weeks for depression	Lundbeck Mylan	IM flupentixol has a mood-elevating effect and is well tolerated at these doses. Extrapyramidal effects are rarely seen. Side effects reported include dry mouth, dizziness, and drowsiness.

CHAPTER 13

Drug	Dosing Information	Manufacturer	Notes
Scopolamine	0.3mg once or twice daily as an adjunct to conventional antidepressants	Generic scopolamine	Very limited evidence; not recommended Anticholinergic adverse effects are common: blurred vision, dry mouth, drowsiness, dizziness, tachycardia, anxiety
Clozapine	Use half the equivalent oral dose	Apotheek A15	Adverse effects are the same as for oral dosing Injection site reactions (pain, nodules) are common if repeated doses are given over several weeks

Subcutaneous

Drug	Dosing Information	Manufacturer	Notes
Haloperidol	Subcutaneous injection ■ 0.5–3mg, max 10mg/day Continuous subcutaneous infusion ■ 0.5–1.5mg/24h, max 10mg/day	Generic haloperidol short-acting injection	Dose depends on indication – see product literature
Olanzapine	Subcutaneous bolus injection ■ 5mg BD – TDS (up to 10mg TDS has been described)[83] Continuous subcutaneous infusion ■ Up to 20mg/24h[84]	Use the short-acting IM preparation	SC olanzapine appears to be well tolerated, but data are limited to case reports in end of life care
Risperidone	Subcutaneous injection every 1–2 months Dose depends on response to oral risperidone – see product literature	Teva Pharmaceuticals (USA)	Does not require loading doses or supplementation with oral risperidone
Fluphenazine	Test dose of 12.5–25mg, followed by doses determined by response. See product literature.	Generic fluphenazine long-acting injection	No longer marketed in some countries
Sodium valproate	Continuous subcutaneous infusion: 500–2500mg/day	Use the intravenous formulation	Data are limited to case series in end of life care

Transdermal

Drug	Dosing Information	Manufacturer	Notes
Transdermal selegiline	6mg/24h, 9mg/24h, 12mg/24h Starting dose is 6mg/24h. Titration to higher doses in 3mg/24h increments at ≥ 2-week intervals, up to a maximum dose of 12mg/24h[101].	Bristol Myers Squib, available via Alliance Wholesaler	The 6mg/24h dose does not require a tyramine restricted diet. At higher doses, although no hypertensive crisis reactions have been reported, the manufacturer recommends avoiding high-tyramine-content food substances. Application site reactions and insomnia are the most common reported side effects.

CHAPTER 13

Drug	Dosing Information	Manufacturer	Notes
Blonanserin	40–80mg/day	Dainippon Sumitomo Pharma (Japan and South Korea)	
Asenapine	3.8mg/24h Dose may be increased to 5.7mg/24h or 7.6mg/24h after 1 week	Noven Therapeutics (USA)	
Rectal			
Amitriptyline	Doses up to 50mg twice daily	Suppositories have been manufactured by pharmacies	Case reports only
Clomipramine	No detailed information available	Suppositories have been manufactured by pharmacies	Case reports only
Imipramine	No detailed information available	Suppositories have been manufactured by pharmacies	Case reports only
Doxepin	No detailed information available	Capsules have been used rectally	Case reports only
Sertraline	Starting dose: a 25mg tablet was placed inside the rectal chamber daily. This was titrated up at 3-day intervals to a maximal dose of 100mg on day 10.	Tablets have been used rectally	Levels at the 100mg steady state dose revealed detectable serum levels of sertraline, but not the metabolite. The levels fell within the reported range of levels for orally administered sertraline. No adverse effects were recorded.
Trazodone	No detailed information available	Suppositories have been manufactured by pharmacies	Rectal trazodone has been used for postoperative or cancer pain control rather than antidepressant activity.
Carbamazepine	125–250mg up to four times daily	Generic carbamazepine	Rectal dose needs to be approximately 25% higher than the oral to provide similar plasma concentrations.
Lamotrigine	100mg single dose given to healthy volunteers	Tablets and orodispersible tablets have been used rectally	No published data of use in clinical practice
Topiramate	200mg tablet crushed and dispersed in 10ml water for rectal administration in healthy volunteers	Tablet has been used rectally	No published data of use in clinical practice
Sodium valproate	Dilute the liquid in a 1:1 ratio with water for rectal administration	Liquid has been used rectally	Has been used to terminate seizures

Drug	Dosing Information	Manufacturer	Notes
Intranasal			
Esketamine	Adults < 65 years old: ■ Week 1–4: 56mg starting dose, then 56–84mg twice weekly ■ Week 5–8: 56–84mg once weekly ■ Week 9 onward: 56–84mg weekly or fortnightly Adults > 65 years old ■ Week 1–4: 28mg starting dose, then 28–84mg twice weekly ■ Weeks 5–8: 28–84mg once weekly ■ Week 9 onward: 28–84mg weekly or fortnightly	Janssen	Pre/post BP monitoring is required. Patients must not eat or drink for 2h before and 30 min after doses. The patient must recline their head by 45° during administration and sniff gently after administration to keep the medicine inside the nose.
Inhalation			
Loxapine	10mg single dose daily	Alexza Pharmaceuticals	Risk of bronchospasm Patient must be able to close their lips around the device, inhale, hold their breath for up to 10 seconds, then exhale.

Availability of all preparations listed varies over time and from country to country.

CHAPTER 13

References

1. Royal College of Psychiatry. Use of licensed medicines for unlicensed applications in psychiatric practice. *BJPsych Bulletin* 2007; 31: doi:10.1192/pb.bp.107.015370.
2. Kuzin, M. *et al*. Body mass index as a determinant of clozapine plasma concentrations: A pharmacokinetic-based hypothesis. *J Clin Psychopharmacol* 2021; 35(3): 273–278.
3. Kurien, M., *et al*. Impact of direct drug delivery via gastric access devices. *Expert Opin Drug Deliv* 12: 455–463, doi:10.1517/17425247.2015.966683 (2015).
4. McIntyre, C. M. *et al*. Medication absorption considerations in patients with postpyloric enteral feeding tubes. *Am J Health Syst Pharm* 2014 Apr 1; 71(7): 549–556.
5. Pakyurek, M. *et al*. Sublingually administered fluoxetine for major depression in medically compromised patients. *Am J Psychiatry* 1999; 156: 1833–1834.
6. Swainson, J. *et al*. Sublingual ketamine: an option for increasing accessibility of ketamine treatments for depression? *J Clin Psychiatry* 2020; 81: 19lr13146, doi:10.4088/JCP.19lr13146.
7. Morgan, P. T. Treatment-resistant depression: response to low-dose transdermal but not oral selegiline. *J Clin Psychopharmacol* 2007; 27: 313–314, doi:10.1097/01.jcp.0000270085.15253.15.
8. Fowler, J. S. *et al*. Evidence that formulations of the selective MAO-B inhibitor, selegiline, which bypass first-pass metabolism, also inhibit MAO-A in the human brain. *Neuropsychopharmacology* 2015; 40: 650–657, doi:10.1038/npp.2014.214.
9. Robbins, B. *et al*. Amitriptyline absorption in a patient with short bowel syndrome. *Am J Gastroenterol* 1999; 94: 2302–2304, doi:10.1111/j.1572-0241.1999.01323.x.

10. Das, A., *et al.* Options when anti-depressants cannot be used in conventional ways. Clinical case and review of literature. *Person Med Psychiatry* 2019; 15–16, 22–27, doi:https://doi.org/10.1016/j.pmip.2019.01.002.

11. Deisenhammer, E. A. *et al.* Intravenous versus oral administration of amitriptyline in patients with major depression. *J Clin Psychopharmacol* 2000; **20**: 417–422.

12. Koran, L. M., Sallee, F. R. & Pallanti, S. Rapid benefit of intravenous pulse loading of clomipramine in obsessive–compulsive disorder. *Am J Psychiatry* 1997; **154**: 396–401.

13. Svestka, J. *et al.* [Citalopram (Seropram) in tablet and infusion forms in the treatment of major depression]. *Cesk Psychiatr* 1993; **89**: 331–339.

14. Baumann, P. *et al.* A double-blind double–dummy study of citalopram comparing infusion versus oral administration. *J Affect Disord* 1998; **49**: 203–210.

15. Pollock, B. G., *et al.* Acute antidepressant effect following pulse loading with intravenous and oral clomipramine. *Arch Gen Psychiatry* 1989; **46**: 29–35.

16. Moukaddam, N. J. *et al.* Intravenous antidepressants: a review. *Depression and Anxiety* 2004; **19**: 1–9.

17. Sallee, F. R., *et al.* Pulse intravenous clomipramine for depressed adolescents: double–blind, controlled trial. *Am. J. Psychiatry* 1997; **154**: 668–673.

18. Bhikram, T. P. *et al.* The Effect of Intravenous Citalopram on the Neural Substrates of Obsessive-Compulsive Disorder. *J Neuropsychiatry Clin Neurosci* 2016; **28**: 243–247, doi:10.1176/appi.neuropsych.15090213.

19. Guelfi, J. D., *et al.* Efficacy of intravenous citalopram compared with oral citalopram for severe depression. Safety and efficacy data from a double-blind, double-dummy trial. *J Affect Disord* 2000; **58**: 201–209.

20. Kasper, S. *et al.* Intravenous antidepressant treatment: focus on citalopram. *Eur Arch Psychiatry Clin Neurosci* 2002; **252**: 105–109.

21. Delic, M. *et al.* Delirium during I.V. citalopram treatment: a case report. *Pharmacopsychiatry* 2013; **46**: 37–38.

22. Sogaard, B., *et al.* The pharmacokinetics of escitalopram after oral and intravenous administration of single and multiple doses to healthy subjects. *J Clin Pharmacol* 2005; **45**: 1400–1406.

23. Konstantinidis, A. *et al.* Intravenous mirtazapine in the treatment of depressed inpatients. *Eur Neuropsychopharmacol* 2002; **12**: 57–60.

24. Muhlbacher, M. *et al.* Intravenous mirtazapine is safe and effective in the treatment of depressed inpatients. *Neuropsychobiology* 2006; **53**: 83–87.

25. Guclu, S., *et al.* Mirtazapine use in resistant hyperemesis gravidarum: report of three cases and review of the literature. *Arch Gynecol Obstet* 2005; **272**: 298–300.

26. Schwarzer, V., *et al.* Treatment resistant hyperemesis gravidarum in a patient with type 1 diabetes mellitus: neonatal withdrawal symptoms after successful antiemetic therapy with mirtazapine. *Arch Gynecol Obstet* 2008; **277**: 67–69.

27. Collins, J. J., *et al.* Intravenous amitriptyline in pediatrics. *J Pain Symptom Manage* 1995; **10**: 471–475.

28. RX List. http://www.rxlist.com, 2021.

29. Koran, L. M., *et al.* Pulse loading versus gradual dosing of intravenous clomipramine in obsessive-compulsive disorder. *Eur Neuropsychopharmacol* 1998; **8**: 121–126.

30. Fiorentini, A. *et al.* Efficacy of oral trazodone slow release following intravenous administration in depressed patients: a naturalistic study. *Riv Psichiatr* 2018; **53**: 261–266, doi:10.1708/3000.30005.

31. Ballerio, M. *et al.* Clinical effectiveness of parenteral trazodone for the management of psychomotor activation in patients with bipolar disorder. *Neuro Endocrinol Lett* 2018; **39**: 205–208.

32. Crapanzano, C., *et al.* Intramuscular and intravenous trazodone for the treatment of agitation. *European neuropsychopharmacology* 2019; **29**: S241, doi:10.1016/j.euroneuro.2018.11.386.

33. Murrough, J. W. *et al.* Antidepressant efficacy of ketamine in treatment-resistant major depression: a two-site randomized controlled trial. *Am J Psychiatry* 2013; **170**: 1134–1142.

34. Lapidus, K. A. *et al.* A randomized controlled trial of intranasal ketamine in major depressive disorder. *Biol Psychiatry* 2014; **76**: 970–976, doi:10.1016/j.biopsych.2014.03.026.

35. Loo, C. K. *et al.* Placebo-controlled pilot trial testing dose titration and intravenous, intramuscular and subcutaneous routes for ketamine in depression. *Acta Psychiatr Scand* 2016; **134**: 48–56, doi:10.1111/acps.12572.

36. George, D. *et al.* Pilot randomized controlled trial of titrated subcutaneous ketamine in older patients with treatment-resistant depression. *Am J Geriatr Psychiatry* 2017; **25**: 1199–1209, doi:10.1016/j.jagp.2017.06.007.).

37. Lara, D. R., *et al.* Antidepressant, mood stabilizing and procognitive effects of very low dose sublingual ketamine in refractory unipolar and bipolar depression. *Int J Neuropsychopharmacol* 2013; **16**: 2111–2117, doi:10.1017/s1461145713000485.

38. Nguyen, L. *et al.* Off-label use of transmucosal ketamine as a rapid-acting antidepressant: a retrospective chart review. *Neuropsychiatr Dis Treat* 2015; **11**: 2667–2673, doi:10.2147/ndt.s88569.

39. Jaffe, R. J., *et al.* Scopolamine as an antidepressant: a systematic review. *Clin Neuropharmacol* 2013; **36**: 24–26.

40. Furey, M. L. *et al.* Pulsed intravenous administration of scopolamine produces rapid antidepressant effects and modest side effects. *J Clin Psychiatry* 2013; **74**: 850–851.

41. Drevets, W. C. *et al.* Replication of scopolamine's antidepressant efficacy in major depressive disorder: a randomized, placebo-controlled clinical trial. *Biol Psychiatry* 2010; **67**: 432–438.

42. Moćko, P., *et al.* The potential of scopolamine as an antidepressant in major depressive disorder: a systematic review of randomized controlled trials. *Biomedicines* 2023; **11**, doi:10.3390/biomedicines11102636.

43. Maragakis, B. P. A double-blind comparison of oral amitriptyline and low–dose intramuscular flupenthixol decanoate in depressive illness. *Curr Med Res Opin* 1990; **12**: 51–57, doi:10.1185/03007999009111491.

44. Gerner, P., *et al.* Topical amitriptyline in healthy volunteers. *Reg Anesth Pain Med* 2003; **28**: 289–293.

45. Ho, K. Y., *et al.* Topical amitriptyline versus lidocaine in the treatment of neuropathic pain. *Clin. J. Pain* 2008; **24**: 51–55.

46. Melero, A. *et al.* Nortriptyline for smoking cessation: release and human skin diffusion from patches. *Int. J. Pharm.* 2009; **378**: 101–107.

47. Sandig, *et al.* Transdermal delivery of imipramine and doxepin from newly oil-in-water nanoemulsions for an analgesic and anti-allodynic activity: development, characterization and in vivo evaluation. *Colloids Surf B Biointerfaces* 2013; **103**: 558–565.

48. Sunderland, T. *et al.* High-dose selegiline in treatment-resistant older depressive patients. *Arch Gen Psychiatry* 1994; **51**: 607–615.

49. Mann, J. J. *et al.* A controlled study of the antidepressant efficacy and side effects of (-)-deprenyl. A selective monoamine oxidase inhibitor. *Arch Gen Psychiatry* 1989; **46**: 45–50.

50. Rossano, F. *et al.* Efficacy and safety of selegiline across different psychiatric disorders: A systematic review and meta-analysis of oral and transdermal formulations. *Eur Neuropsychopharmacol* 2023; **72**: 60–78, doi:10.1016/j.euroneuro.2023.03.012.

51. Viatris. https://www.viatris.com/en-us/lm/countryhome/us-products/productcatalog/productdetails?id=bcd487dc-1180-48d3-a0ca-4ac8927c6 980 . 2021.

52. Wecker, L., *et al.* Transdermal selegiline: targeted effects on monoamine oxidases in the brain. *Biol Psychiatry* 2003; **54**: 1099–1104.

53. Azzaro, A. J., *et al.* Pharmacokinetics and absolute bioavailability of selegiline following treatment of healthy subjects with the selegiline transdermal system (6 mg/24 h): a comparison with oral selegiline capsules. *J Clin Pharmacol* 2007; **47**: 1256–1267.

54. Amsterdam, J. D. *et al.* Selegiline transdermal system in the prevention of relapse of major depressive disorder: a 52-week, double-blind, placebo-substitution, parallel-group clinical trial. *J Clin Psychopharmacol* 2006; **26**: 579–586.

55. Adams, S. Amitriptyline suppositories. *N Engl J Med* 1982; **306**: 996.

56. Mirassou, M. M. Rectal antidepressant medication in the treatment of depression. *J Clin Psychiatry* 1998; **59**: 29.

57. Storey, P. *et al.* Rectal doxepin and carbamazepine therapy in patients with cancer. *N Engl J Med* 1992; **327**: 1318–1319.

58. Chaumeil, J. C. *et al.* Formulation of suppositories containing imipramine and clomipramine chlorhydrates. *Drug Dev Ind Pharm* 1988; **15–17**: 2225–2239.

59. Leung, J. G., *et al.* Rectal bioavailability of sertraline tablets in a critically ill patient with bowel compromise. *J Clin Psychopharmacol* 2017; **37**: 372–373, doi:10.1097/jcp.0000000000000685.

60. Organon Pharma (UK) Limited. Summary of product characteristics – Sycrest 10mg sublingual tablets. 2023.

61. Douzenis, A., *et al.* Sublingual use of olanzapine in combination with alprazolam to treat agitation in a terminally ill patient receiving parenteral nutrition. *Eur J Cancer Care (Engl)* 2007; **16**: 289–290, doi:10.1111/j.1365-2354.2006.00735.x.

62. Bascom, P. B., *et al.* High-dose neuroleptics and neuroleptic rotation for agitated delirium near the end of life. *Am J Hosp Palliat Care* 2014; **31**: 808–811, doi:10.1177/1049909113507124.

63. Markowitz, J. S. *et al.* Pharmacokinetics of olanzapine after single–dose oral administration of standard tablet versus normal and sublingual administration of an orally disintegrating tablet in normal volunteers. *J Clin Pharmacol* 2006; **46**: 164–171, doi:10.1177/0091270005283839.).

64. Yap, R., *et al.* Comfort care kit: use of nonoral and nonparenteral rescue medications at home for terminally ill patients with swallowing difficulty. *J Palliat Med* 2014; **17**: 575–578, doi:10.1089/jpm.2013.0364.

65. Taylor, D. M., *et al.* The Maudsley® Prescribing Guidelines in Psychiatry. 14 edn. Wiley Blackwell, 2021.

66. Lokshin, P., *et al.* Parenteral clozapine: five years of experience. *J Clin Psychopharmacol* 1999; **19**: 479–480.

67. Meltzer, H. Y. Treatment of the neuroleptic-nonresponsive schizophrenic patient. *Schizophrenia Bulletin* 1992; **18**: doi:10.1093/schbul/18.3.515.

68. Munzar, B. *et al.* Clinical experience with intramuscular clozapine. *Cureus* 2021, doi:10.7759/cureus.18267.

69. Kasinathan, J. *et al.* Evaluating the use of enforced clozapine in an Australian forensic psychiatric setting: two cases. *BMC Psychiatry* 2007; **7**: doi:10.1186/1471-244x-7-s1-p13.

70. Schulte, P. F. *et al.* Compulsory treatment with clozapine: a retrospective long-term cohort study. *Int J Law Psychiatry* 2007; **30**: 539–545, doi:10.1016/j.ijlp.2007.09.003.

71. Gee, S., *et al.* Intramuscular clozapine in the acute medical hospital: Experiences from a liaison psychiatry team. *SAGE Open Medical Case Reports* 2021; **9**, doi:10.1177/2050313X211004796.

72. Henry, R. *et al.* Evaluation of the effectiveness and acceptability of intramuscular clozapine injection: illustrative case series. *BJPsych Bulletin* 2020, doi:10.1192/bjb.2020.6.

73. Casetta, C. *et al.* A retrospective study of intramuscular clozapine prescription for treatment initiation and maintenance in treatment–resistant psychosis. *Br J Psych Online* 2020 first.

74. Whiskey, E. *et al.* Resolution without discontinuation: heart failure during clozapine treatment. *Ther Adv Psychopharmacol* 2020; **10**: doi:10.1177/2045125320924786.

75. Andersen, T. H., *et al.* Involuntary treatment of schizophrenia patients 2004–2010 in Denmark. *Acta Psychiatr Scand* 2014; **129**: 312–319, doi:10.1111/acps.12144.

76. McLean, G. *et al.* Parenteral clozapine (Clozaril). *Australasian Psychiatry* 2001; **9**: 371–371, doi:10.1046/j.1440-1665.2001.0367a.x.

77. Gaszner, P., *et al.* Agranulocytosis during clozapine therapy. *Prog Neuro-Psychopharmacol Biol Psychiatry* 2002; **26**: doi:10.1016/S0278-5846(01)00256-1.

78. Schulte, P. F. J. *et al.* Compulsory treatment with clozapine: A retrospective long-term cohort study. *Int J Law Psychiatry* 2007; doi:10.1016/j.ijlp.2007.09.003.

79. Khokhar, M. A. *et al*. Droperidol for psychosis-induced aggression or agitation. *Cochrane Database Syst Rev* 2016; **12**: Cd002830, doi:10.1002/14651858.CD002830.pub3.

80. Williams, A. M. Coadministration of intramuscular olanzapine and benzodiazepines in agitated patients with mental illness. *Ment Health Clin* 2018; **8**: 208–213, doi:10.9740/mhc.2018.09.208.

81. Zaporowska-Stachowiak, I., *et al*. Haloperidol in palliative care: Indications and risks. *Biomed Pharmacother* 2020; **132**: 110772, doi:https://doi.org/10.1016/j.biopha.2020.110772.

82. Tchobaniouk, L. V. *et al*. Once-monthly subcutaneously administered risperidone in the treatment of schizophrenia: patient considerations. *Patient Prefer Adherence* 2019; **13**: 2233–2241, doi:10.2147/ppa.S192418.

83. Elsayem, A. *et al*. Subcutaneous olanzapine for hyperactive or mixed delirium in patients with advanced cancer: a preliminary study. *J Pain Symptom Manage* 2010; **40**: 774–782, doi:10.1016/j.painsymman.2010.02.017.

84. Hindmarsh, J., *et al*. Subcutaneous olanzapine at the end of life in a patient with schizophrenia and dysphagia. *Palliat Med Rep* 2020; **1**: 72–75, doi:10.1089/pmr.2020.0039.

85. Kondasinghe, J. S., *et al*. Subcutaneous levetiracetam and sodium valproate use in palliative care patients. *J Pain Palliat Care Pharmacother* 2022; **36**: 228–232, doi:10.1080/15360288.2022.2107145.

86. Birnbaum, A. K., *et al*. Rectal absorption of lamotrigine compressed tablets. *Epilepsia* 2000; **41**: 850–853.

87. Birnbaum, A. K., *et al*. Relative bioavailability of lamotrigine chewable dispersible tablets administered rectally. *Pharmacotherapy: J Human Pharmacol Drug Therapy* 2001; **21**: 158–162.

88. Anderson, G. D. *et al*. Current oral and non–oral routes of antiepileptic drug delivery. *Adv Drug Deliv Rev* 2012; **64**: 911–918, doi:10.1016/j.addr.2012.01.017.

89. Conway, J. M., *et al*. Relative bioavailability of topiramate administered rectally. *Epilepsy Res* 2003; **54**: 91–96.

90. Carter Snead, O. *et al*. Treatment of status epilepticus in children with rectal sodium valproate. *J Pediatrics* 1985; **106**: 323–325, doi:https://doi.org/10.1016/S0022-3476(85)80318-8.

91. Clemens, P. L., *et al*. Relative bioavailability, metabolism and tolerability of rectally administered oxcarbazepine suspension. *Clin Drug Investig* 2007; **27**: 243–250, doi:10.2165/00044011-200727040-00003.

92. Karlin, D. M., *et al*. Dexmedetomidine sublingual film: a new treatment to reduce agitation in schizophrenia and bipolar disorders. *Ann Pharmacother* 2024; **58** 54–64, doi:10.1177/10600280231171179.

93. Lopes, R., *et al*. The utility of intravenous clomipramine in a case of Cotard's syndrome. *Rev.Bras.Psiquiatr.* 2013; **35**: 212–213.

94. Fallon, B. A. *et al*. Intravenous clomipramine for obsessive-compulsive disorder refractory to oral clomipramine: a placebo–controlled study. *Arch Gen Psychiatry* 1998; **55**: 918–924.

95. Karameh, W. K. *et al*. Intravenous clomipramine for treatment-resistant obsessive-compulsive disorder. *Int J Neuropsychopharmacol.* 2015; **19**: pyv084, doi:10.1093/ijnp/pyv084.

96. Buoli, M. *et al*. Is trazodone more effective than clomipramine in major depressed outpatients? A single-blind study with intravenous and oral administration. *CNS Spectr* 2017; 1–7, doi:10.1017/s1092852917000773.

97. Park, L. *et al*. Neurophysiological changes associated with antidepressant response to ketamine not observed in a negative trial of scopolamine in major depressive disorder. *Int J Neuropsychopharmacol* 2019; **22**: 10–18, doi:10.1093/ijnp/pyy051.

98. Chen, J. C. C. *et al*. A randomized controlled trial of intravenous scopolamine versus active-placebo glycopyrrolate in patients with major depressive disorder. *J Clin Psychiatry* 2022; **83**: doi:10.4088/JCP.21m14310.

99. Beach, S. R., *et al*. Intravenous haloperidol: A systematic review of side effects and recommendations for clinical use. *Gen Hosp Psychiatry* 2020; **67**: 42–50, doi:https://doi.org/10.1016/j.genhosppsych.2020.08.008.

100. Fontana, E. *et al*. Intravenous valproate in the treatment of acute manic episode in bipolar disorder: A review. *J Affect Disord* 2020; **260**: 738–743, doi:10.1016/j.jad.2019.08.071.

101. Nandagopal, J. J. *et al*. Selegiline transdermal system: a novel treatment option for major depressive disorder. *Expert Opin Pharmacother* 2009; **10**: 1665–1673.

CHAPTER 13

Index

The Maudsley® Prescribing Guidelines for Mental Health Conditions in Physical Illness, First Edition.
Siobhan Gee and David M. Taylor.
© 2025 John Wiley & Sons Ltd. Published 2025 by John Wiley & Sons Ltd.